WORLD FOOD AND NUTRITION STUDY

The Potential Contributions of Research

Prepared by the
Steering Committee
NRC Study on World Food and Nutrition
of the
Commission on International Relations
National Research Council

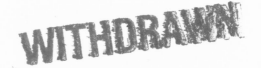

NATIONAL ACADEMY OF SCIENCES
WASHINGTON, D.C.   1977

Library of Congress Catalog Card Number 77-81318
International Standard Book Number 0-309-02628-8

Available from:

Printing and Publishing Office
National Academy of Sciences
2101 Constitution Avenue, N.W.
Washington, D.C. 20418

Printed in the United States of America

June 20, 1977

1977
NOV 4

The President
The White House
Washington, D.C. 20500

My dear Mr. President:

I take great pleasure in transmitting to you a report from the National Research Council entitled *World Food and Nutrition Study: The Potential Contributions of Research.*

Shortly after the World Food Conference in Rome in 1974, President Gerald R. Ford requested the assistance of the National Academy of Sciences in "a major effort to lessen the grim prospect that future generations of peoples around the world will be confronted with chronic shortages of food and with the debilitating effects of malnutrition." Specifically, we were asked to "make an assessment of this problem and develop specific recommendations on how our research and development capabilities can best be applied to meeting this major challenge."

We gladly accepted this invitation, since the prevalence of hunger and malnutrition in the world is a matter of great concern to this Academy as well as to the worldwide community of scientists. A Steering Committee, chaired by Professor Harrison Brown of the California Institute of Technology, was empaneled to conduct this study. They enlisted the assistance of 14 special study teams and, in addition, more than a thousand other knowledgeable individuals, at home and abroad, were given opportunity to contribute their special insights and recommendations.

In November 1975, we transmitted to President Ford the preliminary findings of the Steering Committee as summarized in *Interim Report: World Food and Nutrition Study.* At the same time, we also transmitted the report, *Enhancement of Food Production for the United States,* prepared by our Board on Agriculture and Renewable Resources under the chairmanship of Professor Sylvan Wittwer of Michigan State University.

In your Inaugural Address you made clear that while the United States, alone, cannot guarantee the basic rights of every human being to be free of poverty, hunger, disease, and repression, we can and will

iii

cooperate with others in combating these ancient enemies of human-kind. Whereas overcoming the problems of widespread hunger and malnutrition in the world and greatly increasing food availability at reasonable cost will be extremely complex endeavors, requiring action along many lines, there is reason to be hopeful, nevertheless. This report concludes that, given the political will here and abroad, it should be possible, by the end of this century, to eliminate most of the hunger and malnutrition now associated with mass poverty.

The report indicates that the substantial research and development capabilities and educational resources of the United States can make a major contribution to the world capability to achieve markedly increased food availability and to minimize the age-old threats of hunger and malnutrition. At the same time, these efforts could benefit both the producers and consumers of food in our own country by lowering production costs, increasing agricultural profitability, and helping to contain the rising cost of food.

This report is in three parts. Chapter 1 presents an analysis of the world food and nutrition situation in all of its complexity, and points out the special role that accelerated research and development can play in resolution of the problems. Chapter 2 contains a carefully evaluated listing of the most promising areas of research and development, based upon studies made by 12 teams of experts. Chapter 3 offers recommendations concerning the mechanisms for getting the job done. Specific suggestions are made regarding appropriate responsibilities of the Department of Agriculture, the Agency for International Development, the National Science Foundation, and the Department of Health, Education, and Welfare as well as of other concerned agencies of the federal government. The report emphasizes that, if this program is to succeed, it is particularly important that your office coordinate our national endeavors and develop an international effort commensurate with the need.

In addition to this final report you will shortly receive five volumes containing the full reports of the study teams which undertook the detailed analyses and evaluations. May I take this opportunity to express the appreciation of the Academy to Professor Brown for his inspired leadership of this study, to Dr. Joel Bernstein, the Study Director, for his superb management of this enterprise and to all those who so generously contributed their time and creativity to our common cause. Our thanks are tendered as well to the National Science Foundation, the Department of Agriculture, the Department of Health, Education, and Welfare, the Department of State, and the Agency for

International Development, for their cooperation in and support of this endeavor.

Now that this task has been completed, we want to assure you, Mr. President, that the National Academy of Sciences stands ready to work with you, in any way it can, in a major world effort to free humankind at last from the scourge of hunger and malnutrition.

Sincerely yours,

Philip Handler
President
National Academy of Sciences

WORLD FOOD AND NUTRITION STUDY
STEERING COMMITTEE

Contents

Foreword

Few of the challenges facing humanity are larger or more important than the problem of world hunger and malnutrition.* Why is it that hundreds of millions of our fellow human beings are inadequately nourished? Why is it that, in spite of our technological progress, millions of persons die each year as the direct or indirect result of inadequate food intake? What steps can be taken to lessen the suffering and stress that are the consequences of not having enough to eat?

These and other questions were discussed at the World Food Conference held in Rome in 1974. Shortly thereafter the President of the United States wrote to the President of the National Academy of Sciences asking the Academy to "make an assessment of this problem and develop specific recommendations on how our research and development capabilities can best be applied to meeting this major challenge."

The President's request was accepted and the study was begun in June 1975. This is the final report of the Steering Committee appointed to undertake that study.

Chapter 1 of this report, "Dimensions of the World Food and Nutrition Problem," represents the effort of the Steering Committee to comply with the President's request to make an assessment of the world food

---

* Throughout this report we define "hunger" as a craving or urgent need for food, and "malnutrition" as faulty or inadequate nutrition. Clearly a person can be malnourished without being hungry because either the intake of specific nutrients is too small or too large.

xi

and nutrition situation. The problem, as the Committee makes clear, is a very complex one composed of a number of critical interacting parts. Research and development are shown to be but two of the components (albeit extremely important ones) of an effective program for lessening hunger and malnutrition.

The adequacy of food supplies, of course, is critical, but much more is involved. In particular, widespread poverty in the developing countries is a major cause of hunger and malnutrition. The stability of supplies and prices at local, national, and international levels is an important factor affecting the ability of food systems to meet food and nutritional needs. Government policies are often inappropriate and the organizations serving food systems do not always perform effectively.

The rapid rate of population growth is a contributor to hunger and malnutrition. However, there is growing evidence that improvements in nutrition as well as in education and health are likely to be accompanied by declines in fertility. We propose that the question of just how specific aspects of development affect fertility be an important component of a separate major study on population.

Chapter 2, "High Priority Research," represents the first part of our attempt to comply with the President's request to "develop specific recommendations on how our research and development capabilities can best be applied to meeting this major challenge." Defining "research" as the search for new knowledge and "development" as the application of knowledge to the solution of practical problems, we first attempted to list promising research and development approaches to the solution of the various aspects of the world food and nutrition problem. That listing, which was compiled by a number of study teams, was very long. Using procedures described in Chapter 2, the proposed research areas were then evaluated and from them 22 were selected as containing particular lines of research that would have the greatest effect on world food and nutrition during the next few decades. We believe that these 22 areas should be given the highest priority by the government of the United States, along with other nations.

Chapter 3, "How to Get the Work Done," represents an attempt to examine the research priorities as they relate to national and international institutional arrangements and funding requirements. We emphasize that, while much of the research and development can be undertaken in U.S. institutions, a large part of it must be undertaken in the developing countries. Special attention was given, therefore, to mechanisms whereby research and educational institutions in the United States might most effectively help developing countries expand and strengthen their own research and development capabilities.

The greater part of the work leading to the recommendations in Chapters 2 and 3 was undertaken by 14 study teams. The Steering Committee is deeply grateful to the chairmen and members of the various study teams for their dedicated work, undertaken for the most part under heavy pressure of time. The full study team reports are presented in subsequent volumes of this report. The study teams are responsible for the content of their reports, which were reviewed by the Steering Committee.

Although most of the members of the Steering Committee and of the study teams have had considerable international experience, it nevertheless seemed essential to obtain the views of experts from other parts of the world concerning these problems. Accordingly, four seminars were held—the first in Bangkok, Thailand, with Asian scientists; the second in Cali, Colombia, with Latin American scientists; the third in Nairobi, Kenya, with scientists from Africa and the Middle East; and the fourth near Vienna, with scientists from Eastern and Western Europe. Letters were sent to 200 scientists and administrators in developing countries who are concerned with problems of food and nutrition, seeking their views on issues before the Steering Committee, and many thoughtful responses were received. Many of the views expressed at those seminars and in the letters are incorporated in the recommendations of the Steering Committee.

Numerous other persons were consulted. These included many officials of the sponsoring U.S. agencies and representatives of land-grant and other universities, of development assistance organizations, and of public interest groups. Scientists and administrators of the public and private research communities working on food and nutrition were consulted extensively, as were population experts. Consultations were also held with the Technical Advisory Committee of the Consultative Group on International Agricultural Research, with the directors and deputy directors of many of the international agricultural research centers, and with other international experts.

Five U.S. government agencies gave financial support to this study: the National Science Foundation, the Department of Agriculture, the Department of Health, Education, and Welfare, the State Department, and the Agency for International Development.

As chairman of the Steering Committee, I thank the Committee members for their countless hours of hard work. Above all, I thank the study director, Joel Bernstein, for his dedicated efforts, and other members of the staff who have done so much to make this report possible.

I look upon this report as the beginning rather than the end of a process. It is hoped that it will stimulate a series of actions by the government of the United States that will help to strengthen and extend worldwide efforts aimed at substantially reducing hunger and malnutrition.

HARRISON BROWN, *Chairman*
Steering Committee
World Food and Nutrition Study

Acknowledgments

Approximately 1,500 people have contributed their ideas and comments to this report. It is not possible to list all of their names here, but the Steering Committee is deeply grateful to them.

Study Teams

The largest contribution to this study was made by the 14 study teams listed below. Each team submitted a report in its subject area. These are published separately as *Supporting Papers, World Food and Nutrition Study.* The Steering Committee drew on the contents of these reports and the other ideas and materials generated by the study teams for Chapters 2 and 3 of this report. The Committee is fully responsible for the form in which it has used recommendations and analyses from the study teams.

The study teams other than the priorities panel (Study Team 13) solicited suggestions and comments from appropriate individuals in the scientific community, many of them from developing countries. We are grateful to these experts who made many valuable contributions to this effort.

STUDY TEAM 1 (CROP PRODUCTIVITY)

Richard H. Wellman (*Chairman*), Boyce Thompson Institute for Plant Research
Samuel R. Aldrich, University of Illinois

Frederick Ausubel, Harvard University
John D. Axtell, Purdue University
Glenn W. Burton, U.S. Department of Agriculture
Peter S. Carlson, Michigan State University
Ralph W. F. Hardy, du Pont Company
A. Colin McClung, The Rockefeller Foundation
Woodrow W. McPherson, University of Florida
T. Kelley White, Purdue University
Israel Zelitch, Connecticut Agricultural Experiment Station

Subgroup A (Pest Control)

Ray F. Smith (*Chairman*), University of California, Berkeley
Perry L. Adkisson, Texas A&M University
Boysie E. Day, University of California, Berkeley
John H. Perkins, Miami University
John B. Siddall, Zoecon Corporation
H. David Thurston, Cornell University

STUDY TEAM 2 (ANIMAL PRODUCTIVITY)

Tony J. Cunha (*Chairman*), California Polytechnic State University
James M. Fransen, International Bank for Reconstruction and Development
Harlow J. Hodgson, University of Wisconsin
James E. Johnston, The Rockefeller Foundation
Wilford H. Morris, Purdue University
Robert R. Oltjen, U.S. Department of Agriculture
W. R. Pritchard, University of California, Davis
Kenneth H. Shapiro, University of Michigan
Robert R. Spitzer, U.S. Agency for International Development
N. L. VanDemark, Cornell University

Subgroup A (Animal Health)

W. R. Pritchard (*Chairman*), University of California, Davis
Edward T. Braye, Tuskegee Institute
William M. Moulton, U.S. Department of Agriculture
Philip A. O'Berry, U.S. Department of Agriculture
Calvin W. Schwabe, University of California, Davis

STUDY TEAM 3 (AQUATIC FOOD SOURCES)

John E. Bardach (*Chairman*), Hawaii Institute of Marine Biology and
    East-West Center
Harvey R. Bullis, Jr., National Oceanic and Atmospheric Administration

James A. Crutchfield, Jr., University of Washington
Harold L. Goodwin, Bethesda, Maryland
John E. Halver, University of Washington
Harlan C. Lampe, University of Rhode Island
John C. Marr, Mardela Fisheries, Ltd.
Robert D. May, Hawaii Institute of Marine Biology
George M. Pigott, University of Washington
Eddie W. Shell, Auburn University
Lucian M. Sprague, International Bank for Reconstruction and Development
Kenneth E. F. Watt, University of California, Davis

STUDY TEAM 4 (RESOURCES FOR AGRICULTURE)

Jan van Schilfgaarde (*Chairman*), U.S. Salinity Laboratory, U.S. Department of Agriculture

Subgroup A (Farming Systems)

Edwin Oyer (*Chairman*), Cornell University
Lee R. Martin, University of Minnesota and U.S. Agency for International Development
Donald L. Plucknett, University of Hawaii and U.S. Agency for International Development
Jose Vicente-Chandler, U.S. Department of Agriculture
Frank G. Viets, Fort Collins, Colorado

Subgroup B (Land and Water)

G. R. Stairs (*Chairman*), University of Arizona
William E. Martin, University of Arizona
Arnold C. Orvedal, Lanham, Maryland
Dean Peterson, U.S. Agency for International Development
Pedro Sanchez, North Carolina State University

Subgroup C (Fertilizers)

Lewis Nelson (*Chairman*), Tennessee Valley Authority
Douglas Lathwell, Cornell University
William P. Lockeretz, Washington University
Paul Stangel, International Fertilizer Development Center

Subgroup D (Energy and Equipment)

W. E. Splinter (*Chairman*), University of Nebraska
B. Delworth Gardner, Utah State University
Roy Harrington, Deere and Company

Gary H. Heichel, University of Minnesota and U.S. Department of Agriculture

David Wolf, Sperry–New Holland Company

STUDY TEAM 5 (WEATHER AND CLIMATE)

A formal study team was not established. The recent NAS study, *Climate and Food*, was drawn on heavily for materials in this field and the following consultants were used:

Wayne Decker (Chairman of the committee responsible for *Climate and Food*), University of Missouri

Louis J. Battan, University of Arizona

William C. Burrows, Deere and Company

Ray E. Jensen, National Oceanic and Atmospheric Administration and Texas A&M University

John E. Kutzbach, University of Wisconsin

Richard C. McArdle, U.S. Department of Agriculture

J. Murray Mitchell, Jr., National Oceanic and Atmospheric Administration

STUDY TEAM 6 (FOOD AVAILABILITY TO CONSUMERS)

Carl W. Hall (*Chairman*), Washington State University

Subgroup A (Food Losses)

Philip E. Nelson (*Chairman*), Purdue University
Adolf F. Clausi, General Foods Corporation
Essex D. Finney, U.S. Department of Agriculture
C. Gene Haugh, Purdue University
Abdul R. Rahman, U.S. Army Natick Laboratories

Subgroup B (Food Processing and Preservation)

Bernard S. Schweigert (*Chairman*), University of California, Davis
John V. Luck, General Mills, Inc.
George M. Pigott, University of Washington
Walter M. Urbain, Sun City, Arizona
Daniel I. C. Wang, Massachusetts Institute of Technology

Subgroup C (Food Marketing and Distribution)

Ray Goldberg (*Chairman*), Harvard University
Kenneth R. Farrell, U.S. Department of Agriculture
Kelly M. Harrison, Michigan State University
Jerry T. Hutton, Foremost Foods Company
Edward T. Tyrchniewicz, University of Manitoba

STUDY TEAM 7 (RURAL INSTITUTIONS, POLICIES, AND SOCIAL SCIENCE RESEARCH)

G. Edward Schuh (*Chairman*), Purdue University
John Montgomery, Harvard University

Subgroup A (Policies and Program Planning)

Glenn L. Johnson (*Chairman*), Michigan State University
Walter P. Falcon, Stanford University
Roger W. Fox, University of Arizona
Carol Lancaster, U.S. Office of Management and Budget

Subgroup B (Research, Education and Training, and Extension)

D. Woods Thomas (*Chairman*), Purdue University
George H. Axinn, Michigan State University and Midwest Universities Consortium for International Activities
E. Walter Coward, Cornell University
Alvin A. Johnson, Ithaca, New York
Albert H. Moseman, Ridgefield, Connecticut

Subgroup C (Finance, Input Supplies, and Farmers' Organizations)

Martin E. Abel (*Chairman*), University of Minnesota
Dale W. Adams, Ohio State University
Leon F. Hesser, U.S. Agency for International Development
Bruce F. Johnston, Stanford University
Judith Tendler, Berkeley, California

STUDY TEAM 8 (INFORMATION SYSTEMS)

Ludwig Eisgruber (*Chairman*), Oregon State University
James T. Bonnen, Michigan State University
Richard A. Farley, U.S. Department of Agriculture
Bryant E. Kearl, University of Wisconsin
William E. Kibler, U.S. Department of Agriculture
Robert R. McDonald, National Aeronautics and Space Administration
Ithiel de Sola Pool, Massachusetts Institute of Technology
Bruce Scherr, Data Resources, Inc.
John Woolston, International Development Research Centre, Canada

STUDY TEAM 9 (NUTRITION)

Alan Berg (*Chairman*), International Bank for Reconstruction and Development
James Austin, Harvard Business School

Doris H. Calloway, University of California, Berkeley
Sol Chafkin, The Ford Foundation
Gail Harrison, University of Arizona
Gerald T. Keusch, Mount Sinai Hospital, New York
Jodie Levin-Epstein, The Children's Foundation
Hamish N. Munro, Massachusetts Institute of Technology
E. R. Pariser, Massachusetts Institute of Technology
C. Peter Timmer, Harvard School of Public Health

STUDY TEAM 10 (INTERDEPENDENCIES)

David Pimentel (*Chairman*), Cornell University

Subgroup A (*Population and Health*)

W. Henry Mosley (*Chairman*), Johns Hopkins University
Don E. Dumond, University of Oregon
Nathan Keyfitz, Harvard School of Public Health
T. Paul Schultz, Yale University

Subgroup B (*Energy, Resources, and Environment*)

Bill Stout (*Chairman*), Michigan State University
Arthur S. Boughey, University of California, Irvine
Pierre Crosson, Resources for the Future, Inc.
Richard C. Jordan, University of Minnesota
Eugene P. Odum, University of Georgia

Subgroup C (*International Trade Policy and Comity Between Nations*)

Dale E. Hathaway (*Chairman*), International Food Policy Research In-
    stitute
Donald F. Hadwiger, Iowa State University
T. K. Warley, University of Guelph
Quentin M. West, U.S. Department of Agriculture

Subgroup D (*National Development Policies*)

John P. Lewis (*Chairman*), Princeton University
R. Albert Berry, University of Toronto
John W. Mellor, U.S. Agency for International Development and Cornell
    University
Manning Nash, University of Chicago

STUDY TEAM 11 (NEW APPROACHES TO INCREASING FOOD SUPPLIES)

Gerard Piel (*Chairman*), *Scientific American*
Raymond Altevogt, Greenbelt, Maryland

George Bugliarello, Polytechnic Institute of New York
John R. Calaprice, University of California, Santa Barbara
Elmer L. Gaden, Jr., University of Vermont
Martin Gibbs, Brandeis University
Arthur E. Goldschmidt, New York, New York
Jimmye S. Hillman, University of Arizona
A. Carl Leopold, University of Nebraska
Roger Revelle, University of California, San Diego
Virginia Walbot, Washington University
Marjorie Whiting, Washington, D.C.

STUDY TEAM 12 (NEW APPROACHES TO THE ALLEVIATION OF HUNGER)

Leroy Wehrle (*Chairman*), Sangamon State University
Avrom Bendavid-Val, Center for Growth Alternatives
Al Cardenas, ADM Milling Company
Joseph R. Gusfield, University of California, San Diego
Norge W. Jerome, University of Kansas Medical Center
F. P. Mehrlich, U.S. Army Natick Laboratories
Morris D. Morris, Overseas Development Council and University of Washington
Robert R. Nathan, Robert R. Nathan Associates, Inc.
James Pines, Transcentury Corporation
Richard A. Smith, University of Hawaii School of Medicine and U.S. Department of Health, Education, and Welfare
Victor C. Uchendu, University of Illinois

STUDY TEAM 13 (RESEARCH PRIORITY ASSESSMENT)

Emery N. Castle (*Chairman*), Resources for the Future, Inc.
Aaron M. Altschul, Georgetown University Medical School
Chester B. Baker, University of Illinois
Lawrence Bogorad, Harvard University
Harold E. Calbert, University of Wisconsin
Gerald A. Carlson, North Carolina State University
Robert F. Chandler, Templeton, Massachusetts
Lehman B. Fletcher, Iowa State University
D. Mark Hegsted, Harvard School of Public Health
Keith A. Huston, University of Minnesota
John D. Isaacs, Scripps Institution of Oceanography
James H. Jensen, Green Valley, Arizona
Herbert W. Johnson, University of Minnesota
Robert L. Metcalf, University of Illinois
Harold F. Robinson, Western Carolina University
Lauren Soth, West Des Moines, Iowa
Carl E. Taylor, Johns Hopkins University

K. L. Turk, Ithaca, New York
S. G. Younkin, Campbell Soup Company

STUDY TEAM 14 (AGRICULTURAL RESEARCH ORGANIZATION)

E. T. York (*Chairman*), State University System of Florida
Olle Bjorkman, Carnegie Institute of Washington
Charles V. Kidd, Association of American Universities
Harold F. Robinson, Western Carolina University

Subgroup A (Research Organization in the United States)

Charles Hess (*Chairman*), University of California, Davis
Ronald D. Knutson, Texas A&M University
J. Edward Legates, North Carolina State University
Charles E. Palm, Cornell University

Subgroup B (Global Agricultural Research Organization)

Paul Miller (*Chairman*), Rochester Institute of Technology
Glenn Beck, U.S. Agency for International Development
Dana G. Dalrymple, U.S. Department of Agriculture and U.S. Agency for
    International Development
Lowell S. Hardin, The Ford Foundation
Lewis Perinbaum, Canadian International Development Agency

Subgroup C (Development of Research Personnel)

John Murdock (*Chairman*), University of Wisconsin
Russell G. Mawby, Kellogg Foundation
Hugh Popenoe, University of Florida
A. Russell Stevenson, Agricultural Development Council
Burton Swanson, University of Illinois

The following individuals consulted on the work of the various study teams:
Robert E. Evenson, Agricultural Development Council, Study Team 14;
Walter L. Fishel, U.S. Department of Agriculture, Study Team 13; Jack
Keller, Utah State University, Study Team 4; and C. Richard Shumway,
Texas A&M University, Study Team 13.

Staff

We are especially indebted to the staff of this study for their perseverance
and diligent efforts. The professional staff are: Joel Bernstein, Study Director;

Sabra Bissette (August 1976–publication); Ruth L. Emerson; Charles E. French; Charles E. Hanrahan; Kenneth F. Harling (July 1975–March 1976); and Barbara West (May 1975–August 1976). The support staff are: Brenda Buchbinder, Gerard E. Hoyt, Gray Mason, Rosena Ricks, and Zenaida G. Scott.

Valuable part-time staff assistance was received from other staff members of the Commission on International Relations: professional help from Jay J. Davenport, Julien Engel, John G. Hurley, and W. Murray Todd; support staff help from Yvonne Cassells, Betty Green, Suzanne M. Lavender, and Roberta Ross. Assistance was also received from Robert C. Rooney and Cecilia Larsen of the Commission on Natural Resources.

This report was edited by Robert R. Hume, Executive Editor of the National Research Council, and Barbara Davies, a consulting editor.

Other Academy Personnel

The members of the Board on Agriculture and Renewable Resources made large contributions to the study over the period August 1975 to March 1976 by discussion and review of draft materials. Members of the Food and Nutrition Board made contributions in the same way. Suggestions were also made by members and staff of the Commission on International Relations and of the Division of Biological Sciences of the Assembly of Life Sciences. Finally, many useful suggestions were received from an Academy report review committee: Vincent P. Dole, Rockefeller University; Robert McC. Adams, University of Chicago; Richard L. Garwin, IBM Corporation; Sterling B. Hendricks, Silver Spring, Maryland; Jay L. Lush, Iowa State University; Frederick Mosteller, Harvard University; Kenneth B. Raper, University of Wisconsin; Charles M. Rick, Jr., University of California, Davis; Theodore W. Schultz, University of Chicago; Frank W. Westheimer, Harvard University; Gilbert F. White, University of Colorado; and Saunders MacLane, University of Chicago, overall chairman of the Academy's report review process.

International Contributions

The Steering Committee is particularly indebted to the groups of foreign experts that met with Steering Committee representatives in Thailand, Kenya, Austria, and Colombia to discuss issues connected with the study. The individuals who are listed below made significant contributions to the study, but they do not necessarily agree with any particular conclusions or recommendations: Resat Aktan, University of Ankara, Turkey; Julio A. Andrews, Asia Foundation, The Philippines; D. S. Athwal, International Rice Research Institute, The Philippines; Antonio Bacigalupo, Food and Agriculture Organization, Colombia; D. F. R. Bommer, Food and Agriculture Organization,

Italy; Francisco Cardenas Ramos, Instituto Nacional de Investigaciones Agricolas, Mexico; Charan Chantalakhana, Kasetsart University, Thailand; Yung Kyung Choi, Office of Rural Development, Korea; C. Choudary, Food and Agriculture Organization, Syria; Luis B. Crouch, Dominican Republic; J. D. Drilon, Jr., Southeast Asian Regional Center for Graduate Study and Research in Agriculture, The Philippines; Salah El-Zarka, Food and Agriculture Organization Regional Fisheries Office for Near East and Africa, Egypt; Alexander Grobman, Centro Internacional de Agricultura Tropical, Colombia; A. F. Gurnett-Smith, Commonwealth Scientific and Industrial Research Organization, Australia; Yujiro Hayami, Tokyo Metropolitan University, Japan; Diego Londono, Instituto Colombiana Agropecuari, Colombia; C. L. Luh, Asian Vegetable Research and Development Center, Republic of China; Joseph C. Madamba, Philippine Council for Agriculture and Resources Research, The Philippines; B. N. Majisu, East African Agriculture and Forest Research Organization, Kenya; D. Menasveta, Southeast Asia Fisheries Development Center, Thailand; Moise N. Mensah, Consultative Group on Food Production and Investment, Washington, D.C.; Fernando Monckeburg, University of Chile: Agide Gorgatti Netto, Instituto de Tecnologia de Alimentos, Brazil; Mohamed A. Nour, Food and Agriculture Organization Regional Representative for the Near East, Egypt; Thomas R. Odhiambo, International Center for Insect Physiology and Ecology, Kenya; Bede N. Okigbo, International Institute of Tropical Agriculture, Nigeria; Stephan A. Pieniazek, Research Institute of Pomology, Poland; R. E. Pierre, Caribbean Agricultural Research and Development Institute, West Indies; Ferenc Rabar, International Institute for Applied Systems Analysis, Austria; Lucio G. Reca, Argentina; Max Rutman, Ingenieria en Nutricion y Alimentos, Chile; Sanga Sabhasri, National Research Council of Thailand; Mariano Segura-Bustamante, Ministry of Agriculture, Peru; Howard Steppler, MacDonald College, Canada; W. P. Ting, Malaysian Agricultural Research and Development Institute, Malaysia; Yoash Vaadia, Ministry of Agriculture, Israel; Alberto Valdez, International Food Policy Research Institute, Washington, D.C.; Jose Alencar Carneiro Viana, Federal University of Minas Gerais, Brazil; V. S. Vyas, Asian Development Bank, The Philippines; Ray Wijewardene, International Institute of Tropical Agriculture, Nigeria; and D. De Zeeuw, Ministry of Agriculture and Fisheries, The Netherlands.

To supplement the international consultations, the Steering Committee sent a list of questions discussed at the conferences to experts in many parts of the world and received responses from the following: Enrique P. Ampuero, Instituto Nacional de Investigaciones Agropecuarias, Ecuador; M. Behar, World Health Organization, Switzerland; C. F. Bentley, The University of Alberta, Canada; Ricardo Bressani, Instituto de Nutricion de Centro America y Panama, Guatemala; Yen-tien Chang, National Taiwan University, Republic of China; Rubens Vaz da Costa, Brazil; Ralph W. Cummings, Jr., International Agricultural Development Service, New York; S. C. Hsieh, Asian Development Bank, The Philippines; Yoshimaru Inouye,

Asian Productivity Organization, Japan; Yoshiaki Ishizuka, Hokkaido University, Japan; Peter R. Jennings, The Rockefeller Foundation, New York; A. S. Kahlon, Punjab Agricultural University, India; J. S. Kanwar, International Crops Research Institute for the Semi-Arid Tropics, India; Yoshisuke Kishida, Shin-Norinsha Company, Ltd., Japan; H. Mirheydar, Ministry of Agriculture and Natural Resources, Iran; A. Mitra, Jawaharlal Nehru University, India; Hussein Omari Mongi, Uyole Agricultural Center, Tanzania; Amir Muhammed, University of Agriculture, Pakistan; Jose Pastore, University of Sao Paulo, Brazil; Vernon W. Ruttan, Agricultural Development Council, Singapore; A. M. El-Tabey Shehata, University of Alexandria, Egypt; Ernest W. Sprague, International Maize and Wheat Improvement Center, Mexico; D. Sundaresan, National Dairy Research Institute, India; M. S. Swaminathan, Secretary to the Government of India; R. J. Sybenga, Agricultural University, The Netherlands; Allen D. Tillman, The Rockefeller Foundation, Indonesia; K. Vas, Food and Agriculture Organization, Austria; B. H. Waite, University of Florida; Robert Orr Whyte, Institute of Southeast Asian Studies, Singapore; and Don Winkelmann, International Maize and Wheat Improvement Center, Mexico.

Substantial contributions were also received in several group meetings and individually from members of the Technical Advisory Committee of the Consultative Group on International Agricultural Research (CGIAR); the directors, deputy directors, and principal economists of nine of the international agricultural research centers located in developing countries that are supported by CGIAR; and the directors of the International Fertilizer Development Center (Alabama), the Asian Vegetable Research and Development Center (Taiwan), the International Food Policy Research Institute (Washington), and the Tropical Products Institute (London). The staffs of the International Maize and Wheat Improvement Center in Mexico and the International Rice Research Institute in the Philippines provided much material on the international research collaboration and training in which those centers are involved.

Documentation and other assistance also were contributed by the secretariat of CGIAR, the World Bank staff, the Ford Foundation, the Rockefeller Foundation, the Population Council, and the Food and Agriculture Organization of the United Nations.

Federal Agencies

Extensive assistance was received from research administrators and staff from the following U.S. government agencies: Department of Agriculture, Agency for International Development, National Science Foundation, National Institutes of Health and other agencies within the Department of Health, Education, and Welfare, National Oceanic and Atmospheric Administration, State Department, Office of Management and Budget, Tennessee

Valley Authority, and the Office of Science and Technology Policy. Representatives of several of these agencies met with the Steering Committee and provided documents, critiques of issues and ideas, and responses to questions. Other valuable inputs resulted from staff participation in a series of conferences and meetings on research issues sponsored by the Agricultural Research and Policy Advisory Committee to the Secretary of Agriculture, which is jointly operated by the Department of Agriculture and the land-grant universities.

Useful inputs also were received from several congressional sources: from staffs at the Office of Technology Assessment and the Library of Congress, and from informal comments made by members of the Senate and the House of Representatives.

Private Organizations

Many contributions were made by the administrators and staff of U.S. universities involved in food and nutrition research and of other private research organizations, and by staff and officers of the university associations, particularly the National Association of State Universities and Land Grant Colleges. Similarly, extensive comments were received from research managers of many U.S. companies. Public interest groups contributed other comments and suggestions. Useful inputs also resulted from staff participation at an international conference at Harbor Springs, Michigan, on research imperatives for increasing crop productivity, which was jointly sponsored by the agricultural experiment station at Michigan State University and the Charles F. Kettering Foundation.

Summary

1. *Dimensions of the World Food and Nutrition Problem*

The world food system is not working adequately for either poor or rich countries. Large and increasing numbers of people are hungry and malnourished. Associated with hunger are other matters of increasing seriousness: rising costs of food production, unstable market conditions, and increasing evidence that the content of diets is a major contributor to health problems in virtually all countries, including the United States.

Human beings suffer from several kinds of malnutrition. They can be harmed by eating too little food, or too much food, or by the wrong amounts or balance of particular elements in their diet. These types of malnutrition are found in all countries, but undernourishment is particularly widespread in the poor countries, while the other kinds of malnutrition are prominent in rich countries like the United States.

Possibly as many as 450 million to a billion persons in the world do not receive enough food. Most of the hungry people live in the poor countries where populations are destined to grow rapidly for some time into the future.

Since World War II, the growth of population and of total income in most of the world has been unprecedented, and this has further increased demands for food. World population grew 60 percent from 1950 to 1975; 80 percent of this growth was in the developing countries. From 1950 to 1974, the gross national product (GNP) per person in both the developing and the high-income countries more than doubled.

1

It is likely that by the turn of the century per capita GNP will have doubled again.

The immediate cause of hunger is the lack of resources with which to buy or produce enough food. Insufficient food interacts with disease, apathy, and other effects of poverty to foster malnutrition and lower productivity. Thus such problems as the inequitable distribution of income and unemployment are important aspects of the problem of world hunger.

Sharp fluctuations in world food supplies and prices aggravate problems of hunger and malnutrition. The variability in production due to weather, pests, and disease, and government policies to stabilize internal prices contribute to the instability of food prices and supplies.

Another important cause of malnutrition is the absence or weakness of policies, institutions, and programs to foster the best use of available food supplies for the purpose of improving nutrition. In poor and rich countries alike, governments, private organizations, and individuals continually make decisions that affect nutritional status with little or no knowledge of the nutritional consequences.

The most important requirement for the alleviation of malnutrition is for the developing countries to double their own food production by the end of the century. We are convinced that this can be done given the political will in the developing and higher-income countries.

Thus the problem of alleviating hunger and malnutrition in the world is a complex one. Success will depend upon how effectively we undertake four major tasks: increasing the supply of the right kinds of food where it is needed, reducing poverty, improving the stability of food supplies, and decreasing the rate of population growth.

INCREASING FOOD SUPPLY

If the developing countries are to increase per capita food availability by at least 1 percent per year, they need to expand their food production over the next 25 years at an average rate of about 3 to 4 percent per year. How much of the increase in food supply will be available to increase per capita consumption will depend on how fast the rate of population growth declines.

Expanding crop area and increasing crop production per hectare are the two ways to increase food production. Increases of crop area probably will not exceed an average of 1 percent per year over the next 25 years and may be appreciably less. Thus increases in yield need to average about 2.5 percent per year. This will not be easy to achieve and sustain, but it is encouraging that the developing countries collectively increased their food production by 38 percent during the period

1965 to 1975. Major efforts, organized around improved farming technologies, will be needed to achieve the necessary rates of increase.

This situation also will create pressures upon the United States to increase food production at an appreciable rate. Our population is still growing. Further, if the developing countries continue to import increasing amounts of their food from the United States, and if the import demands of Europe and Japan continue to rise because of growing affluence, increased U.S. productivity will be necessary to reduce rising pressures on U.S. food prices and production costs. This necessitates finding ways to increase our agricultural yields still further.

REDUCING POVERTY

Two essential conditions for reducing poverty in the developing countries are rapid expansion of employment and an increased supply of food. Maximum use of the available work force simultaneously expands output and personal incomes, particularly at the lower end of the income scale. Expanding food supply fulfills the principal consumption needs of the poor at a lower cost and promotes the growth of national income. Simultaneously expanding national employment, food supply, and the well-being of workers depends heavily on introducing more productive technologies throughout the food system that make better use of workers. Direct food distribution programs can help alleviate poverty and correct the maldistribution of food.

STABILIZATION OF FOOD SUPPLIES

Local, national, and international measures are needed to prevent sudden drops in food supplies, market gluts that discourage production, and sharply fluctuating food prices. Improved technology can reduce food losses caused by weather and pests. Appropriate government policies also can reduce instability in food supplies and prices. And national and international arrangements for food reserves can remedy cycles of glut and shortage.

POPULATION GROWTH

In the short run, gains in nutrition in low-income countries may increase population growth rates by decreasing mortality before fertility declines. However, there is evidence that the social and economic changes required for increased food production and better health also are conducive to reduced birth rates.

In the long run, no action is more important for improving the world food and nutrition situation than the reduction of birth rates. In view of this fact, *we strongly recommend that the U.S. government sponsor a study to assess how U.S. research capabilities can best be applied to help countries desiring effective means of reducing birth rates.*

THE ROLE OF RESEARCH AND DEVELOPMENT

A strong research base is essential to all activities needed to increase the food supply, reduce poverty, and moderate the instability of supplies and prices. The role of research is to broaden the range of choices available to all those who affect world food supply and nutrition such as farmers, consumers, and government officials. In stressing this we do not assume that research and development will solve world food problems, only that it is an essential part of the solution.

A broad spectrum of research and development activities, ranging from adaptation of existing technologies to the search for new scientific discoveries, is necessary to improve the performance of food systems. In this study we particularly stress the need for biological innovations, improved farming systems, improved technologies aimed at reducing risks, and improved development policies and organizations. We also emphasize research that concentrates on the effects of malnutrition. Finally, we stress the great importance of expanding basic food and nutrition research. Many of the improvements we visualize cannot be brought about unless our reservoir of relevant basic knowledge is enlarged.

THE ROLE OF THE UNITED STATES

The United States, along with other high-income nations, can contribute to the solution of problems of hunger and malnutrition by providing capital assistance, cooperating in the formulation of development plans, and working for a more effective international environment in trade and the management of food reserves. Larger U.S. involvement in these activities is desirable.

The United States can play a very important role in research and development. Our experience in research and in the training of research workers could help the developing countries build their own research capabilities. This is particularly important because many problems can be studied only in the environments in which they occur. Programs of a large number of research and educational institutions in the United States could be redesigned to include more studies of selected world food and nutrition problems.

The effect that research efforts by the United States could have on world food problems depends on the extent and quality of U.S. working relationships with national and international research organizations in the developing countries.

RECOMMENDATIONS

In the light of our analyses, we recommend: (1) expanded research efforts to improve food and nutrition policies, increase food availability, reduce poverty, and stabilize food supplies; (2) actions to help mobilize and organize research and development resources in the United States and throughout the world; and (3) a U.S. government mechanism to better interrelate actions that affect food and nutrition situations both at home and abroad.

AN OPPORTUNITY

The challenge to U.S. research capabilities that is presented by world food problems is attended by many reasons for optimism.

Our most important reason for optimism is the increasing ability of many developing countries to address their own food problems. Many developing countries have made important progress in addressing the poverty and population growth factors that underlie malnutrition. In addition, the potential for improving agricultural yields in developing countries is clearly very large.

If there is the political will in this country and abroad to capitalize on these promising elements, it should be possible to overcome the worst aspects of widespread hunger and malnutrition within one generation. By the end of the century, grain production could be doubled in the developing countries and food production in the rich countries could be increased by more than the total grain production of the United States today.

We find these prospects exciting and worthy of strong national and international efforts.

2. High Priority Research

HOW PRIORITIES WERE ESTABLISHED

The selection of major research areas and promising approaches for achieving them was based on their prospective effects on world hunger over the next few decades.

To establish priorities, 12 interdisciplinary study teams were assembled and asked to identify research and development areas with outstanding potential to help meet world food and nutrition needs. Three questions posed by the Steering Committee guided the selection of these areas:

– What advances in knowledge will specific areas of research produce, and what is the scientific or technological significance of these advances?
– If the research produces results, what effect would they likely have on reducing global hunger and malnutrition over the next several decades?
– What supportive action will be required to conduct research for the accelerated activity recommended (e.g., more resources, policy changes, organizational changes)?

The priority areas identified by the study teams, which totaled over 100, were then evaluated by Study Team 13, which examined the important areas from a number of points of view, including near-term effects (less than 15 years) and longer term effects (more than 15 years). This ranking resulted in the designation of 22 priority areas. They were selected because of the likelihood that important advances toward the broad goal of each research area were feasible and would contribute significantly to improving the world food and nutrition situation. Particularly promising individual lines of research are identified within each priority area. The 22 selected priority research areas fall into four categories: nutrition, food production, food marketing, and policies and organizations. Some recommended priority lines of research promise possible widespread application within 5 to 10 years. Others will produce results only over the longer term. No rankings are made among the 22 areas; they constitute the minimum of a highly selected list of promising types of research requiring support.

• *We recommend that U.S. research support be increased for the lines of research identified within these 22 research areas:*

• Nutrition–Performance Relations
• Role of Dietary Components
• Policies Affecting Nutrition
• Nutrition Intervention Programs
• Plant Breeding and Genetic Manipulation
• Biological Nitrogen Fixation
• Photosynthesis

- Resistance to Environmental Stresses
- Pest Management
- Weather and Climate
- Management of Tropical Soils
- Irrigation and Water Management
- Fertilizer Sources
- Ruminant Livestock
- Aquatic Food Sources
- Farm Production Systems
- Postharvest Losses
- Market Expansion
- National Food Policies and Organizations
- Trade Policy
- Food Reserves
- Information Systems

NUTRITION

Nutrition is fundamental to human life, performance, and well-being. This report discusses priorities for various parts of the food system; however, all priorities are based on the goal of adequate nutrition for all segments of the world population.

There is little systematic examination of the effects on human populations of national and international policies affecting nutrition. In this connection, research is needed not only on the extent and functional significance of malnutrition, but also on the merit of present and future policies affecting nutrition. Specifically, we propose research on:

- how present diets affect human functional performance;
- what foods can best meet nutritional needs under differing circumstances;
- government policies that indirectly affect nutrition;
- how best to reach people through programs for improving the nutritional status of particular population groups.

Improved diets can be a major factor in enhancing human well-being. Changes in diet may well turn out to be beneficial to the health and life expectancy of large segments of the population in the United States. In the developing countries, effective nutrition interventions are likely to have more of an effect on human health than comparable investments in medical care.

FOOD PRODUCTION

Research on food production can find the technical means for improving yields and stability of yields of the most important food plants. The low-income countries of the tropics particularly face difficult problems in achieving self-sustaining farming systems that produce high, stable yields with a minimum dependence on energy and capital. During this century, scientific advances have extended our ability to develop new crop and animal strains tailored to the needs of particular regions or special uses. Among the more obvious examples are high yielding hybrid corn and sorghum and the semidwarf varieties of wheat, rice, and barley. We suspect we are nowhere near the natural limits of plant productivity. New techniques of genetic manipulation will permit us to achieve much greater productivity in the future.

Plant Breeding and Genetic Manipulation   Research support should be increased in three areas: revitalizing work on the "classical" genetics and plant breeding methodology of economic plants; work at the cellular level aimed at producing preconceived genetic changes and the development of methods to screen for agronomically important traits; and improving genetic stocks. This work requires collaboration among scientists in this country and abroad who are working in classical genetics and plant breeding, cell biology, and related fundamental scientific fields.

Biological Nitrogen Fixation   Nitrogen is a critical element in protein and therefore in the growth of plants and animals. The large increases in yields over the past 25 years, particularly in the high-income countries, have resulted from the increased use of nitrogen fertilizers. Even so, two-thirds to three-fourths of the nitrogen fixed in association with world agriculture is estimated to occur biologically: microorganisms extract it from the air and fix it in soils and plants. The greater use of this source of nitrogen for plant growth is a reasonable prospect and should be a prime research goal.

Shortages of natural gas and petroleum and the rising costs of the raw materials used to produce chemical fertilizers are persuasive reasons for accelerating research on biological alternatives. Moreover, such research is likely to be useful in reducing the environmental contamination associated with chemical fertilizers.

There are several promising lines of research for increasing biological nitrogen fixation. These include identifying and improving the symbiotic associations between leguminous plants and microorganisms, inducing a similar association between microorganisms and cereal grains, and transferring the genetic capability for nitrogen fixation directly from bacteria to plants.

If cereal crops could fix nitrogen at 30 percent of the soybean rate, the additional nitrogen fixed would equal 36 million tons. This amount of nitrogen is more than five times the total amount currently used in the developing countries.

Photosynthesis Perhaps the greatest potential for using the sun's energy lies in increasing the efficiency with which crops fix solar energy through photosynthesis. Most plants capture no more than 1 to 3 percent of the solar energy they receive. What we know presently indicates a theoretical conversion potential of about 12 percent. Experts suggest that increases in the photosynthetic efficiency of plants could produce gains of 50 percent to well over 100 percent in agricultural yield after 15 years of intensive research.

Resistance to Environmental Stresses The principal causes of instability of food output are stresses on plants such as pests, weather aberrations, and chemical variations in soils. Notable in the latter case are aluminum toxicity and related nutrient deficiencies of acid soils, and salinity.

We assign high priority to several areas of research to reduce the vulnerability of crops to stress, including steps to identify, screen, and breed resistant plants.

Pest Management The losses from pests are known only imprecisely but, worldwide, they may average a third of potential production. Rice, the world's most important crop, suffers losses of perhaps 40 to 50 percent.

Three areas of research should have high priority: the use of agronomic practices to control pests (the foundation of improved pest management systems), breeding for resistance to plant pests, and the introduction of organisms that prey on particular pests.

Weather and Climate Fluctuations in weather and climate cause the largest variations in food production. World food reserves are insufficient to compensate for harvest losses due to the serious weather fluctuations that could occur in a single year. Thus efforts to alleviate problems arising from droughts, unseasonably high or low temperatures, and severe storms are crucial.

We give highest priority to two related areas of research. Our first priority recognizes that agriculture must make better use of weather and climate information. Research to this end would have three objectives: better use of statistical techniques for estimating weather and climate changes; development of more sophisticated models for handling farm risks; and improved management skills for dealing with the effects of weather variability. The second priority is research to improve the analytical techniques for predicting the effects of weather on crops, recognizing that, in large part, agriculture must adapt to the variability of weather and climate.

Management of Tropical Soils   Most of the potentially arable land that is not farmed is in the tropics of Africa and South America, about 1 billion hectares or three-fourths again as much land as is presently cultivated in the world. Seventy percent of this unused arable land has acidic soil belonging to the groups called oxisols and ultisols. There are encouraging indications that these two soil types, if handled properly, can produce high crop yields. However, growing conditions in many tropical areas are far from ideal, and much research will be required before cultivated crops can be grown economically and without affecting the environment adversely.

The sequence of recommended research includes: classifying local soil types, establishing suitable land-clearing methods, identifying methods to correct deficiencies in soil composition which could be used in combination with new stress-resistant plant varieties, identifying measures to enhance water retention and root penetration, developing suitable cropping systems and/or forage-animal systems, and adapting technologies to local ecologic and socioeconomic conditions.

Annual crop production in these humid lands, if well-managed, could be raised to 150 to 200 percent of the temperate zone production per hectare.

Irrigation and Water Management   Adequate water is indispensable for plant growth. Having enough water depends not only on average annual precipitation, but also on the reliability of supply. Farming systems can be highly productive on relatively small annual supplies, if the supplies are dependable or if the soil adequately stores water in relation to variations in rainfall. Unfortunately, precipitation is the most variable and least predictable element of weather.

Today, 14 percent of the world's farmed area is irrigated, and estimates suggest that the area irrigated could be more than doubled. However, as most of the world's farmers will not have access to irrigation, there is also a great need for improved water management in rainfed agriculture.

The recommended research priorities stress improving onfarm water management, supplemented by research and development on physical improvements and on new planning techniques to guide farmers.

Fertilizer Sources The use of chemical fertilizers is usually the most rapid means of increasing farm production. As we have seen, research on biological nitrogen fixation deserves high priority worldwide, but research on inorganic chemical nutrients also is needed.

Two research efforts are recommended to develop new sources of fertilizers: one is for less expensive methods of fixing nitrogen that do not use the increasingly scarce supplies of natural gas and petroleum, the principal raw materials for current production. The other is for the design of fertilizers that can be efficiently used in the tropics.

Other research includes the expanded use of rock phosphates and the use of larger percentages of phosphate ores, better provision for applying micronutrients that are important in the tropics, and the development of slow-release fertilizer.

Ruminant Livestock Animal products are a major part of the world's diet and could play a more important role in the developing countries. In the United States, different types of livestock supply two-thirds of the protein for human consumption. In the developing countries, animal products are a much smaller but still important part of the diet, providing 20 percent of the protein for human consumption. However, animal production has been rising rapidly and can increase severalfold in the future if research and development can overcome certain obstacles.

Two-thirds of the world's agricultural land is in permanent pasture, range, and meadow, of which 60 percent is not suitable for cultivation. These lands, where not claimed for other uses, are exploited best by large ruminant livestock, primarily beef and dairy cattle, which now produce almost half of the world's meat products and most of its milk products. Animals constitute an important stockpile of food and capital for the developing countries. The total caloric worth of worldwide animal stocks in 1974 was 50 percent more than that of grain stocks, and the animal stocks were more evenly distributed.

Animal yields can best be increased by three lines of research: improving feed supply from forage plants in the open ranges and other pasture situations; improving animal health by concentrating on the most damaging contagious diseases; and increasing the offspring of animals that best use low quality diets and resist disease.

Aquatic Food Sources Fish are an important component of total human and animal food intake. In 1974, the world commercial production of food products from fresh and saltwater was about 70 million tons, excluding whales and seals. Five million tons were obtained from aquaculture, mostly in freshwater.

Fisheries and aquaculture differ. Fisheries are essentially gatherings of wild animals, whereas aquaculture employs varying degrees of direct animal management. The application of research to increase production of aquatic animals holds promise in both areas. Research for fuller use of the fish catch could produce early results that would benefit both the United States and the developing countries. It is estimated that the amount of fish protein directly consumed by humans could be doubled without increasing the present world catch.

Research on aquaculture will lead to greater yields. The annual yield of pond fish in Southeast Asia could be increased fivefold from the present average of 600 kilograms per hectare through polyculture coupled with the development of nutrition. This technical potential, combined with the developing countries' growing interest in aquaculture, promises substantial gains.

Genetic improvements will permit the larger-scale gains needed in the long run. Fish geneticists estimate that gains in production from selective breeding alone could soon amount to 2 to 5 percent per year.

Farm Production Systems   The use of new technologies by farmers in the developing countries is inhibited because technology usually comes to them, if at all, in disconnected pieces. Thus they have difficulty fitting it effectively into their farming and social systems. Research on the structure of those systems is of high priority. Since farming systems comprise many factors, this research must be multidisciplinary.

Research on farm production systems has excellent prospects for greatly increasing production, income, and social well-being. It should include:

— selecting crop combinations for the best total income and nutrition;
— introducing improved varieties of crops and animals that permit higher yields, increased annual production per farm, and more stable incomes through adjustments in the length, timing, and mixture of growing seasons;
— preserving the diversity of species and protecting soil resources for long-term production;
— experimenting with crop combinations, sequences, and improved cultivation techniques;
— designing equipment to meet the needs of small farmers for tillage and other cultivation, irrigation, food storage, and crop handling;

– improving the organization and administration of local services;
– improving the management skills of farmers and housewives needed
  for the production, preservation, and consumption of food.

Food production on currently farmed land in the humid tropics can
be increased, perhaps by as much as fourfold in the long run. The introduction of new farming systems requiring minimal inputs of resources
should be important in this regard.

FOOD MARKETING

The quantity and quality of food available to consumers depend upon
a chain of connecting services that determines how well the whole food
system works. The chain can be very short, involving only the farmer
and household members; or it can be long, as in the complex marketing
services of high-income countries.

To improve the quantity and quality of food actually eaten in the
developing countries and also the real income of both producers and
consumers, a number of improvements are needed in these services:

– reduction of waste, which typically is very large;
– reduction of costs;
– better maintenance of food quality, or enhancement by fortification
  or other processing;
– wider and more even distribution of supplies over time and space;
– better communication of consumer demands to producers.

It is estimated that in some parts of the world as much as 50 percent
of the food supply from plants and animals is lost between harvest
and consumption, especially in the humid tropics. The most immediate
research need is to inventory the amount, location, and cause of food
losses. Efforts should then be made to determine whether these causes
are attributable to poor management, inappropriate pricing and policy,
or lack of needed technology.

We recommend the following lines of research as especially promising: extending preharvest pest control to the postharvest phase, and
improving food preservation technologies and storage for the humid
and arid tropics, particularly for use at the farm and village levels.

Markets in the developing countries must be expanded to provide
incentives for increased production, to give consumers a wider variety of
foods at lower cost, and to reduce the food losses that occur when excess
supplies cannot reach markets. One remedy is to expand the purchasing

power of the consumer, especially of the poor consumer. A second remedy, applicable at any level of national income and purchasing power, is to expand the number of markets for farmers in the developing countries.

Research is recommended on means of increasing the purchasing power of poor people in the developing countries: increasing the efficiency of food distribution programs, pricing policies, and product promotion and design. The research needed to expand markets in the developing countries includes: improving transportation; improving intermediate marketing institutions; and adapting modern analytical techniques to the planning, organization, and management of major commodity systems.

The large size of the food sector in the economies of the developing countries and the fact that most of the costs involved in food losses occur after the food leaves the farm suggest that food savings could be considerable.

POLICIES AND ORGANIZATIONS

Science and technology alone cannot improve the world food and nutrition situation. Government policies and the organizations affecting food must provide incentives and opportunities for increased production and better distribution of food. Hence research on social and economic policy is essential.

Illustrations of the effects of national policies and organizations are plentiful. Technology that permits farmers to grow more food at a lower cost per unit of output can be offset by government price, tax, or trade policies that influence the prices of farm products and inputs. These policies can make increased production unprofitable for producers, thereby discouraging use of the new technology. Inadequate credit and marketing services affect the dependability of supplies of seeds, fertilizers, and machinery, and may discourage farmers from applying improved technologies.

International policies and organizations are critically important to the world's food supply. Poor countries would have more incentive to apply better technology in food production if they had better opportunities to expand sales into international markets.

The list of policy and organizational problems is long, and the specific content and relative importance of each differs according to time and place. Experience suggests that the individual developing countries often have common problems regarding their policies and organizations affecting food. Thus it is desirable to develop a number of widely applicable generalizations through comparative analysis of experiences in different countries. However, the size and difficulty of the research needed on policies and organizations require a large increase in current social science research capabilities, both in the United States and in the developing countries.

The developing countries depend upon international trade in food, and upon the principal commodities used to produce food such as fuel, fertilizers, and pesticides, to provide adequate food supplies for their people. The trade policies of both the developing and the high-income countries affect the abilities of the developing countries to meet their national goals.

There are many unknowns about the nature and extent of the interactions among the principal factors affecting trade. These unknowns limit the abilities of individual countries to make rational choices on trade policies and they impede productive dialogue on the international issues. Research is needed to better understand patterns of world food production and trade that take advantage of the resources indigenous to certain areas and that will reflect the real costs of food production in various parts of the world. Research also is needed to permit anticipation of technology and development trends and their implications.

Food reserves are an important means of ensuring the stability of food supplies. Most food stocks are grains, which can be stored and transported more easily than other foods. World grain markets are affected by the interactions of supply, demand, and stocks at national and international levels, and these relationships must be considered when establishing policies for the management of grain stocks.

One line of research would investigate the storage systems of particular developing countries—where stocks are held, who owns stocks, the losses during storage in various types of storage facilities, and the costs and gains from storage. Research should first more accurately describe and evaluate current systems and then evaluate how these systems could be improved.

Another line of research would examine the alternatives to holding grain reserves. For example, international trade may be a feasible alternative for achieving market stabilization and improved distribution. The extent to which food aid could be used to help the developing countries stabilize their food supplies needs to be investigated.

Decision makers need timely information to assess the likely effects of alternative decisions. Decision makers in the developing countries are often severely handicapped by a lack of data. For all countries, policies, programs, and research are becoming more diverse and complex year by year, and requirements for information expand correspondingly.

The developing countries have many information problems and requirements that are similar to those of the high-income countries, although the data required and the complexity of the systems are less. The developing countries already spend sizable portions of their scarce resources on information needs. The information is often unused, either because the wrong data are collected or because there is no way to disseminate the data. Appropriate research can help prevent both problems.

Promising new technology is rapidly being developed to improve information systems. This includes analytical systems for appraising the variables affecting food production, marketing, and nutrition; computer technology; and the capabilities for remote sensing. We can expect a growing number of low-cost systems for use by the developing countries.

Research is recommended on: the information needs of the producer, crop monitoring systems, international data bases for land and nutrition, and total information systems design.

3. *How to Get the Work Done*

Our analysis leads to three major conclusions:

First, a large part of the research needed will have to be carried out in the developing countries, where the most serious shortages of resources for food and nutrition exist. Consequently, the capacity of the developing countries for research and its application must be substantially enlarged.

Second, the international food and nutrition research centers and programs established in tropical countries over the last decade require continued strengthening.

Third, a large part of the research needed will have to be carried out in the high-income countries, where most of the relevant scientific resources are found. In order to undertake its share effectively, the United States should enlarge and reshape its research on food and nutrition.

These objectives need to be approached in combination, not separately, building working relationships among research groups in the high-income and developing countries and the international centers.

RESEARCH CAPACITY IN THE DEVELOPING COUNTRIES

The capacity of the developing countries to conduct research and development on food and nutrition varies substantially from country to country, but all are far short of the scientific and technical resources they need. Those countries must provide the resources they need to build research capacity, but much can be contributed by others, including the United States. We conclude that the United States should, when asked:

- train researchers for the developing countries at U.S. universities and help build training institutions abroad;
- help the developing countries establish research facilities and institutions and apply research results;
- encourage and support communication and collaboration among research workers in the developing countries, in the international and regional institutions, and in the United States on problems of common interest.

INTERNATIONAL RESEARCH CENTERS AND PROGRAMS

Perhaps the largest research contributions to reducing world hunger in recent years have been made by the international agricultural research centers such as the International Rice Research Institute in the Philippines. These centers have produced important research results, have become important training locations, and have contributed to building research capacity in a number of the developing countries. Such centers and programs have a great deal of potential, and they need to be continued and strengthened.

The United States should:

- continue to provide 25 percent of the funding for the centers and programs sponsored by the Consultative Group on International Agricultural Research;
- join in supporting other high quality international centers, both those with which it is already involved and others for which it is not now a major supporter;
- move vigorously and imaginatively to encourage collaborative relationships between international centers and research groups in the United States.

U.S. RESEARCH ON FOOD AND NUTRITION

U.S. research on food and nutrition should enable future U.S. food production and distribution to meet domestic needs at reasonable prices while permitting the continued export of major amounts of food. The research also should contribute to increasing food production and improving food distribution in the developing countries.

Specifically, we conclude that:

- major increases are needed in fundamental research in the natural and social sciences, particularly in those areas related to the enhancement of food production and nutrition;
- a new and broader approach is needed for research on nutrition;
- much greater attention needs to be given by the U.S. research community to international objectives;
- support for social science research relevant to food and nutrition should be increased sharply.

RECOMMENDATIONS FOR U.S. ACTIONS

The Federal–State System of Agricultural Research

Our first set of recommendations concerns the federal–state agricultural research system and the role of the Department of Agriculture (USDA). We consider these recommendations to be the most important we are making on organization and financing. They are intended to enable the Department of Agriculture, in cooperation with other groups, to make a much larger contribution to reducing world hunger and malnutrition than they have thus far. The Department of Agriculture and others involved in agricultural research will need to emphasize and support the entire spectrum of research related to food. They will need to mobilize scientific resources that have not previously been involved with agricultural research. They will need to add to their traditional focus on the United States a direct concern with hunger and malnutrition overseas. Thus the Department of Agriculture and others must develop a substantial and sustained international orientation. Further, they must work in close collaboration on food and nutrition problems with the Agency for International Development.

• *We recommend the appointment of an Assistant Secretary of Agriculture with responsibility only for research and education.*

The Assistant Secretary should be a senior scientist of sufficient stature to attract the highest quality scientific participants.

• *We recommend substantial increases in federal funding for the traditional USDA research programs (including support for state programs), and we recommend funds to establish a new program of competitive grants for research on food and nutrition.*

Increased funding will provide new vitality for the existing system and a stronger base for the accelerated research we recommend.

• *We recommend a first-year increase on the order of $120 million, something under 20 percent of the total of about $700 million of* USDA *and state funds now devoted to food and nutrition research. We propose that the new funds be divided equally between the existing federal–state channels and the new competitive grants program. Thereafter, we recommend successive increases, after adjustments for inflation, on the order of $60 million or approximately 10 percent per year in real terms for the next four years, also divided evenly between the existing programs and the new competitive grants program.*

There is no doubt that funding increases on this scale are needed to attack the larger research agenda and to overcome the effects of the relative neglect of agricultural research in recent decades.

Three points are worthy of note. First, a substantial share of the increased funds will be needed to expand U.S. personnel. Second, we urge that a major new emphasis be placed on nutritional research by the Department of Agriculture. Third, we emphasize the importance of establishing a strong competitive grants program in the Department of Agriculture.

• *We recommend a five-year federal matching grants program for nonfederal research facilities and equipment. These grants should be available to other universities and private nonprofit institutions as well as to those in the land-grant group.*

A large infusion of resources is needed for altering and replacing existing obsolete facilities. Additional facilities will be needed to carry out the proposed research agenda, including a few wholly new installations. Federal funds as large as $100 million per year might be well used.

We reemphasize that Department of Agriculture funds should be used to enable the U.S. scientific community concerned with food and nutrition to become involved in international efforts: to join in collaborative research with colleagues abroad, to conduct research overseas, to undertake training and postdoctoral fellowships in research centers abroad, and to invite foreign scientists to work at U.S. research facilities.

In our view, the Secretary of Agriculture speaks not just for the interests of American food producers but also for the broader interests of all American citizens.

Agency for International Development

Our recommendations propose substantial increases in the scale of and improvements in the substance of the activities of the Agency for International Development (AID) to: help establish research and development capacity in the developing countries, support further development of international research centers and programs, and support U.S. groups that wish to undertake food and nutrition research in the developing countries. Title XII of the Foreign Assistance Act of 1975 provides a new legislative base for these activities and for the participation of U.S. universities in them.

In recent years, AID has suffered a serious deterioration in its professional staff concerned with agriculture, and must rebuild its past competence. The resources of the universities cannot be mobilized and applied to the needs of the developing countries unless there is a high quality professional cadre in AID.

- *We recommend a larger and more systematic effort by* AID *to help the developing countries establish research and development capabilities for food and nutrition in both the natural and social sciences.*

AID has been committing about $30 million per year for this purpose. In our view, that figure should be at least tripled as rapidly as possible.

- *We recommend a larger and better-designed* AID *effort to train research personnel for the developing countries.*

Such an effort should have two main components. The first involves work with U.S. universities to improve the quality and relevance of their training for foreign students. The second involves helping to establish research training programs in the developing countries themselves.

- *We recommend the establishment of a joint* AID–*university committee on international training under Title XII of the Foreign Assistance Act.*
- *We recommend continuation of* AID *support for international research centers and programs, both those supported by the Consultative Group on International Agricultural Research and others of worldwide*

*or regional scope that are likely to provide research results that are
badly needed by the developing countries.*

International research centers involve special risks but they also provide special opportunities. Such centers can contribute significantly to
the build-up of research capacity in the developing countries. To
achieve the potential advantages it is desirable to limit such centers
and programs to those few that are clearly of unusual promise and to
assure their working relationships with national centers in all parts of
the world. U.S. contributions to those centers, which amount to about
$20 million per year and are scheduled to rise by about $4 million per
year over the next several years, are clearly money well spent.

• *We recommend that* AID *enlarge significantly its support for establishing operating relationships between U.S. research groups and those
in the developing countries.*

In recent years, the U.S. universities' knowledge of conditions in
the developing countries, and their direct involvement in those countries, have been declining. We commend the concept, now being developed under Title XII, of support for research programs linking U.S.
and overseas researchers interested in a common problem, such as
adapting soybean cultivation to tropical conditions.

Other forms of support also should be considered. AID should not
hesitate to support research with middle-income countries such as Brazil
or Mexico. Such countries offer some of the best opportunities for
valuable and relatively inexpensive exchanges of research.

Finally, AID should provide encouragement for good university
planning and management of international research. The universities,
in turn, should recognize that the aim of Title XII is to help the developing countries primarily by supporting work there.

National Institutes of Health

The National Institutes of Health (NIH) is the largest source of federal
support for research on human nutrition, spending about $60 million
per year. Most of this research is oriented to the interrelationships between diets and diseases prevalent in the United States.

• *We recommend that* NIH'S *support for nutrition research be reoriented to place greater emphasis on studies of human subjects, par-*

ticularly using epidemiologic approaches and behavioral and other social science skills.

• *We recommend that more effective arrangements be established for coordinating research on nutrition supported by the several Institutes and by other relevant agencies in the Department of Health, Education, and Welfare.*

• *We recommend only modest increments in the* NIH *budget for nutrition research for the immediate future. Some funds from lower priority programs should be diverted to high priority purposes. In the longer run we have no doubt that larger funds will be required.*

National Science Foundation

The central mission of the National Science Foundation (NSF) is to nurture the health of science and the increase of basic knowledge. Support for basic research related to food and nutrition concerns is relatively modest—about $40 million. Large and sustained increases are needed to enlarge as rapidly as possible the stock of fundamental knowledge on which future applied research will depend.

• *We recommend that the National Science Foundation substantially increase its support of fundamental research in biology and other natural science disciplines underlying work on food and nutrition.*

• *We also recommend strengthened support by* NSF *for disciplinary research in the social and behavioral sciences relevant to food and nutrition.*

• *We recommend that funding increases be complemented by increasing the size and duration of individual project financing.*

The authorizing legislation for NSF for fiscal year 1977 places special emphasis on international scientific collaboration to assist in resolving critical world problems such as those of food and population.

• *We recommend vigorous action by* NSF *under this new mandate to promote international scientific collaboration.*

The fiscal year 1977 authorizing legislation also puts new stress on training in interdisciplinary research, including research grants.

• *We recommend that a program of training in interdisciplinary research be undertaken because of its potential for dealing with food and nutrition problems.*

Privately Supported Research

Currently, roughly half of U.S. research and development concerned with food and nutrition is financed in the private sector. Most of this activity is in business firms representing a wide range of industrial pursuits.

• *We recommend that* AID *enlarge its use of contracts to draw on the capacity of private companies to contribute to research and research training objectives in the developing countries.*
• *We also recommend that the Department of Agriculture consider the possibility of making greater use of private resources, by contract, for needed aspects of food and nutrition research where that may bring effective results at equal or smaller public cost.*

Two factors may inhibit the usefulness of normal market-oriented research and development by private business. The first is the possibility that government regulations established in the interest of health, safety, environmental protection, and other purposes may, through overlapping, imprecision, or shortcomings, result in unnecessary or unwise limitations on research and development.

• *We recommend that coordination and simplification of regulations affecting research and development on food and nutrition be given early attention.*

A second set of problems involves patent rights. Issues being raised in international forums challenge the validity, and therefore the effectiveness, of patents and other proprietary rights. There are other prospective problems concerning the adequacy of patent laws as these apply to research on plants.

• *We recommend an early evaluation of U.S. and international proprietary rights under the leadership of the Executive Office of the President.*

Executive Office of the President

It is necessary to establish in the Executive Office of the President arrangements for designing and implementing a coherent strategy for research on food and nutrition. Such a strategy can be established only within the framework of a coherent general strategy for dealing with world food and nutrition problems. We think the operational authority, funds, and programs should be retained in the various departments and agencies. At the same time, a central capacity is needed to look ahead at overall problems.

There are various organizational alternatives for achieving these ends. The essential characteristics are capable leadership and an independent staff.

 • *We recommend the establishment of these two entities in the Executive Office of the President: one to develop and maintain a coherent U.S. strategy for dealing with world food and nutrition problems; the other, subordinate to the first, to facilitate coordination of U.S. and international research activities on food and nutrition.*

1 Dimensions of the World Food and Nutrition Problem

Introduction

Large and increasing numbers of people are hungry and malnourished, but a restless world strongly believes that much of this hunger can be eliminated. The rising costs of food production in many countries threaten higher food prices at a time when the capacity to produce food is seriously underutilized, especially in the poor countries. The world food system could be made to work more effectively for both the poor and the rich countries.

If hunger and malnutrition are not to be the fate of increasing numbers of the world's population, the United States must use its capacities for research and development to counter the rising costs of food production, to reduce the instability of food supplies and prices, and to improve the production capacity and incomes of farmers in the developing countries, many of whom have small land holdings, often in remote areas. Less apparent, but important, is the growing evidence that the content of diets is a significant factor in the health problems of all countries, including the United States. If U.S. research capabilities are used more effectively and supported adequately, they can better serve U.S. needs and contribute more to alleviating world hunger and malnutrition. We believe that the U.S. scientific community is ready and able to undertake this task.

Experience has demonstrated that research that offers new prospects for the food-deficit developing countries can benefit producers and con-

25

sumers both here and abroad. Moreover, unless the productivity of agriculture is increased in the developing countries, the United States may face higher costs of food production and higher food prices for consumers.

This report offers recommendations on how the U.S. scientific community can best serve U.S. and world food needs. As background for these recommendations, we will first examine the food and nutrition situation in the world today.

THE EXTENT AND NATURE OF MALNUTRITION

There is abundant evidence that large numbers of human beings suffer from malnutrition. Estimates by the Food and Agriculture Organization (FAO) and the World Bank, respectively, suggest that around 450 million and possibly as many as a billion people do not receive sufficient food. Most of these people live in the developing countries.

Malnutrition causes millions of premature deaths each year. It is a contributing factor to diseases in many parts of the world, ranging from schistosomiasis in Africa to some kinds of cancer in the United States. In some societies, 40 percent of the children die before they reach the age of five, mostly from nutrition-related causes. A substantial portion of the survivors suffer handicaps of learning, behavior, and work capacity because of inadequate diets and recurring illness.

Concepts regarding the nutritional state of people in the United States are currently being revised. Millions of Americans are overweight to a degree that interferes with their health and longevity. Other health disorders are thought to result from the nature of our food. Possible links between nutrition and diet and the degenerative diseases, learning disabilities, and certain forms of cancer and of mental illness are creating concern in government and scientific circles about the damage being done by malnutrition and about the limitations in our knowledge of nutrition.

Public perceptions of world nutrition problems are conditioned largely by newspaper and relief agency reports about the threat of starvation for millions resulting from disasters such as droughts or floods. Starvation and pockets of severe, chronic food deficiency can and should be virtually eliminated by effective local action, reinforced as needed by help from abroad.

Nutrient deficiencies that cause widespread disease and debilitation chronically affect far more people and cause greater cumulative damage than outright starvation. Malnutrition shortens life expectancy. Acute and chronic infections and anemia reduce work output and induce debility. This loss of vitality undermines a person's capacity to savor life, and the human condition is degraded.

Although hunger and malnutrition have plagued people throughout history, the current situation differs from those of the past. First, with the rapid growth of the world population, the absolute number of malnourished people has increased greatly, although the proportion has decreased. Second, and even more important, a significant segment of human society has learned how to provide itself with enough food by applying scientific knowledge to food production and distribution. That segment, which includes the United States and other high-income countries, has demonstrated conclusively that research, combined with other measures, can contribute substantially to increasing the supply of food, improving its distribution, and enhancing nutrition.

COUNTRY VARIATIONS AND INTERDEPENDENCE

Food problems vary among countries and are generally related to each country's stage of economic development.

The high-income countries, with a gross national product (GNP) per capita in 1975 of about $4,500, include about 1.1 billion people of North America, Europe, Japan, and Oceania. These countries have large numbers of underfed people, but their greatest nutrition problems are caused by the poor quality of diets and overeating.

The middle-income developing countries (excluding the People's Republic of China) include about 800 million people in Asia, Africa, and Latin America with a GNP per capita in 1975 of about $950. This group of countries has the highest rate of population growth (about 2.8 percent annually) because their death rates have dropped far more rapidly than their birth rates. These countries have experienced rapid economic growth and large increases in food production. However, because of population growth and poor income and land distribution in many of these countries, tens of millions remain seriously underfed. Large portions of these populations also suffer from the types of malnutrition that are common in the high-income countries.

The poorest countries, with GNP per capita under $200, include about 1.2 billion people in 36 extremely poor nations spread across Asia and the middle of Africa. Hunger and malnutrition are the most severe in these countries. An estimated one-third to one-half of the people in these countries are malnourished. The lowest-income developing countries provide the least amount of food per person, and currently have the most limited capabilities for increasing production per person and for financing imports.

China and the other centrally planned Asian countries are a fourth group and include an estimated 900 million or more Chinese and residents of the former North Vietnam and of North Korea. Their GNP per capita is probably in the lower range of the middle-income developing countries. Because we lack reliable information on population and food in these countries, the extent of malnutrition is not known with certainty. Many observers report, however, that overt malnutrition is not common. It is important to learn more about the extent and nature of this apparent achievement in dealing with the problem.

Our research recommendations are expected to benefit countries in all four groups, although distinctions are made at some points in our analysis. The recommendations recognize that efforts to improve food supply and nutrition in the United States, in the developing countries, and in the other high-income countries are highly interdependent.

All countries depend on one another to serve as export markets or sources of imports or both: for food products; for supplies or services needed to produce food such as fertilizer, equipment, pesticides, weather information, and credit; or, further back in the food production chain, for petroleum, steel, or technical education. The policies that individual countries or groups of countries pursue to secure markets or sources of supply affect the trade of other countries and the stability of their food supplies and prices. Large-scale changes in population growth and in diet in some parts of the world affect food availability and markets for the other parts. International cooperation can reduce the instability of national food supplies due to weather and pests, and can improve national access to the world's technology and to natural resources used for food production. In light of all these considerations, few countries can be self-contained in meeting their food and nutrition needs. Some might come close to autonomy, but at high cost.

THE PRINCIPAL PROBLEMS OF DEVELOPING COUNTRY AND U.S. FOOD SYSTEMS

In the developing countries, the inadequacy of food systems is principally measured by the serious damage that malnutrition inflicts on their populations. Chronic food shortages and distributional problems are aggravated periodically by bad weather, severe price instability, and the high cost of fertilizer and other production inputs. Incentives to raise the low productivity of food systems and to expand production often are weak.

To eliminate widespread malnutrition, the developing countries must roughly double food production by the end of the century, provide the poorest people adequate access to food supplies, and learn how to provide a healthier diet for all their people. These are difficult but attainable goals.

The U.S. food system has its own performance problems. Food prices have become more unstable, creating uncertainty for both producers and consumers. Price instability is intensified in the United States and in the developing countries by trade barriers and regulated markets in many parts of the world and by the relative weakness of worldwide mechanisms for stabilizing the prices of agricultural commodities. Growing but unstable demand from abroad for U.S. commodities increases the prospect of instability (see Figure 1).

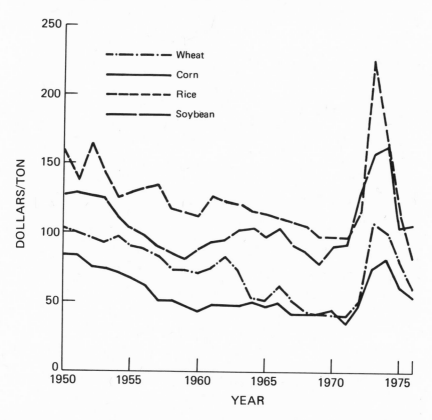

FIGURE 1   U.S. farm-level prices in constant U.S. dollars, 1950–1976. From U.S. Department of Agriculture, Economic Research Service.

Several danger signals portend rising production costs for food in the years ahead unless research and development make possible significant increases in agricultural productivity. These signals include an apparent leveling of yields for major crops (Figure 2), rising costs of energy inputs for all segments of the food system, and loss of land due to wind

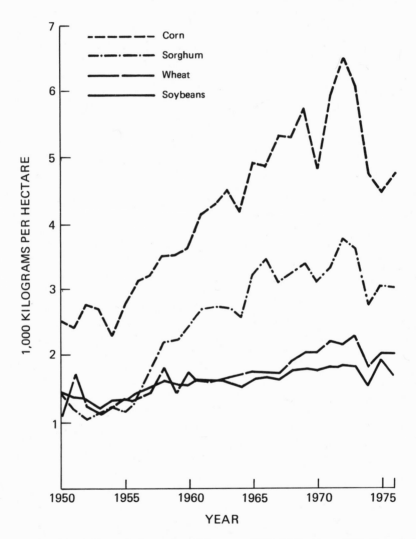

FIGURE 2   Yield trends for major U.S. crops, 1950–1976. From U.S. Department of Agriculture, Economic Research Service.

and water erosion and salinization of irrigated land. Environmental restraints imposed upon the use of agricultural chemicals may increase production costs and result in greater variability in output.

Much of the gain in U.S. agricultural yields and food output since World War II has resulted from large increases in the use of fertilizers, pesticides, equipment, buildings, irrigation systems, and other capital. The prospect of higher costs for energy-intensive farm inputs and of decreasing returns from additional uses requires greater use of other means of increasing yields in order to limit cost increases for farmers and higher food prices for consumers. Greater reliance must be placed on new varieties of crops, improved species of livestock, and farming systems that produce more food from given levels of expenditure on physical inputs.

Farming systems that rely more on biological innovations such as biological nitrogen fixation and pest-resistant and stress-resistant species and less on capital-intensive purchased inputs such as fertilizers, pesticides, and machinery would benefit farmers in the rich and poor countries, including especially poor farmers and farm laborers.

IMPLICATIONS FOR FOREIGN TRADE

Technological gains and the expanded output associated with them can lead to increased specialization in the United States and in the developing countries in those commodities for which each has the greatest cost advantage and to reciprocal increases in imports. Trade policies that permit these gains will benefit producers and consumers in both the United States and the developing countries. Although each country must continue to produce most of its own food, rising consumption levels make it desirable to expand reciprocal trade. The chief gain from imports for the developing countries will be in the lower costs of grain staples. Imports will benefit the United States primarily by increasing the variety in our diets and reducing costs of off-season and tropical fruits and vegetables and other products.

Reciprocal increases in food imports mean expanded exports for the United States and some developing countries. Exports are an important factor in stimulating rapid overall development in the low-income countries.

Food exports also are important to the United States. They provided 21.5 percent of our export earnings from 1971 to 1975. During that period, the United States exported almost 60 percent of its wheat, over 50 percent of its soybeans, and almost 20 percent of its corn. A large and growing commercial market for U.S. agricultural exports exists in low-income countries that achieve rapid agricultural and economic development.

U.S. agricultural exports to the developing countries increased about 400 percent from 1967 to 1976 while the increase to high-income countries was about 240 percent. In 1976, U.S. exports were $11.2 billion to the developing countries and $13.6 billion to the high-income countries. A U.S. Department of Agriculture (USDA) study of 66 countries from 1957 to 1964 showed that, as per capita incomes rose 10 percent, agricultural imports increased 25 percent in low-income countries, 11 percent in medium-income countries, and 8 percent in high-income countries. An analysis of nine developing countries, with a history of rapid development and with annual agricultural production growth substantially faster than that of the United States, showed that their commercial imports of U.S. farm products increased from $56 million in 1955 to $2,469 million in 1973.

Foreign Competition

Expanding agriculture in the developing countries is sometimes thought to conflict with the competitive interests of U.S. agriculture. But as we have seen, U.S. agriculture should benefit greatly from that expansion. Although overseas producers could become competitors of the United States in some commodity markets, the anticipated demand growth accompanying increased agricultural productivity and output will minimize, if not eliminate, the adverse effects upon U.S. producers.

Experience has shown that the worst response that the United States could make to such competitive pressures would be to shield our agriculture from competition. The United States has a large stake in maintaining open world markets for agricultural commodities. New U.S. trade restraints encourage similar measures elsewhere and reduce the markets for U.S. agricultural products. Trade restrictions also remove incentives for cutting costs in U.S. agriculture, thereby damaging our ability to compete and raising food prices for U.S. consumers. A far better course is to make suitable provisions for federal help in easing adjustment problems that may arise.

MUTUAL GAINS

The problems of the U.S. and developing country food systems are highly interrelated. By financing and supporting research to increase the quantity and quality of the world food supply, the United States could benefit in five major ways:

- more profitable farm production and increased incentives to expand production, by countering the rising costs of food production;
- increased supplies of food at reasonable prices, which would help control inflation;
- longer-term markets for exports and sources of low-cost imports for food and other commodities, by stimulating productivity and economic growth in the developing countries;
- reduction of environmental degradation associated with increased use of chemicals in agriculture;
- conservation of scarce petroleum and natural gas used to produce fertilizers and energy for food production.

The Causes of Hunger and Malnutrition

GROWTH OF POPULATION AND OF NATIONAL INCOME

In the two centuries prior to World War II, the rate of population growth gradually increased worldwide. Overall population growth in the developing countries reached an annual rate of increase of about 1 percent. This rate was somewhat slower than in the high-income countries but was characterized by higher birth and death rates. Since World War II, the world population has expanded much faster, especially in the developing countries, primarily because death rates have decreased more rapidly than birth rates. From 1950 to 1975, the world population grew from 2.5 billion to 4 billion persons. Eighty percent of this growth was in the developing countries where rates of population increase rose to an average somewhat over 2.5 percent per year. This rapid growth apparently is beginning to slow down, and may now be 2.3 to 2.4 percent, reflecting declines in birth rates in Asia (including China). Meanwhile, population growth rates in the high-income countries have declined to about 0.7 percent.

Estimates for the future suggest, even with immediate and successful efforts in family planning, a world population of close to 6 billion people by the end of the century unless there is an unwanted increase in mortality. About 90 percent of the additional 2 billion people will be in the developing countries.

In addition to the population growth since World War II, an unprecedented growth of national income in most of the world has increased the demand for food. Average real GNP per person rose about 120 percent in the high-income countries between 1950 and 1974, and about 110 percent in the developing countries, from 1950 levels of about

$2,100 and $170, respectively (at 1973 price levels). Before World War II, the developing countries were net exporters of grains, their principal food. After the war, rising demand exceeded production increases and the developing countries became net importers.

These countries are trying to sustain high growth rates for output and income over the years ahead so that social progress can outpace population growth. This effort will continue the pressure of rising income on food supplies. At the same time, in the high-income countries increasing affluence even with slow population growth is likely to increase the demand for food and feed imports, particularly in Europe and Japan. If food production growth rates should fall below recent levels because of adverse weather or difficulties in increasing productivity in agriculture, affluence and the greater purchasing power of the richer countries will make it very difficult for the poorest nations and poorest people to obtain adequate food supplies.

To contend with these prospects, in addition to the existing food shortages, the developing countries urgently need to expand food supplies more rapidly and distribute them more efficiently over the rest of this century. The high-income countries also will need to expand food production and trade.

POVERTY

The major immediate cause of hunger is poverty. Poverty is the lack of resources with which to buy or produce enough food. Insufficient food in turn combines with disease, apathy, and other effects of poverty to foster malnutrition and lower human productivity.

Poverty exists everywhere, but its extent in a considerable number of countries is massive. The World Bank estimates that 750 million people in the poorest nations live in extreme poverty with annual incomes of less than $75. Even in the middle-income developing countries, World Bank estimates show about 170 million people at the extreme poverty level and hundreds of millions of others are subsisting at income levels less than one-third of their national averages. Most of the extreme poverty is due to low national output and income, combined with maldistribution of the income that is available.

Although food supply has grown slightly faster than population since 1960 in the developing countries as a whole, rapid population growth and inequitable income distribution apparently have combined to increase the absolute numbers of malnourished while the proportion of malnourished has decreased.

INSTABILITY OF FOOD SUPPLY

Sharp fluctuations in food supplies and prices have seriously aggravated the problems of hunger and malnutrition in many parts of the world. Much of the instability arises from acts of nature, such as extreme weather variations or heavy infestations of pests and diseases that destroy crops and animals.

Between 1966 and 1972, the introduction of high yielding food production technologies in the developing countries, accompanied by generally good weather, increased per capita food supplies and created a surge of optimism about reducing world hunger problems. In the next few years, international prices for food products were extremely variable after more than a decade of stability. Production variability, reflecting bad weather, was responsible for part of the price instability. U.S. policies and those of many other governments, which stabilized internal prices by offsetting local production shortfalls with increased imports or decreased exports, also contributed to sharp fluctuations in world food prices.

Favorable weather conditions helped improve crops in 1975 and 1976, but without altering long-term trends indicating the need for greater production efforts, particularly in the developing countries. These improvements, therefore, do not lessen the need to ensure against instability of food supplies in the future. The world food system is still subject to natural and political destabilizing events, and there are few years in which some areas do not experience heavy losses from bad weather or pests.

Price and supply instability have their greatest effect on producers and consumers who are poor and lack the nutritional, food, or financial reserves to endure periods of shortage. In periods of glut, sharply declining prices slash the incomes of poor farmers who cannot afford to hold their crops until prices rise again.

LACK OF A NUTRITION POLICY

Malnutrition is widespread both in countries where food is scarce and in countries where food is plentiful. This suggests that reducing malnutrition depends not only on increasing overall food supply and stabilizing national food supplies, but also on reducing the number of people below poverty income levels, and on improving dietary practices through education and other interventions. This in turn points to the need for governments to give greater attention to the nutritional effects of the full range of their programs and policies.

Governments, private organizations, and individuals continually make decisions and take actions that affect nutritional status with little or no knowledge of the nutritional consequences. Yet few if any countries are systematically working to discover, collect, and apply comprehensive knowledge about the nutritional effects of policies or programs. The extent of malnutrition could be greatly reduced with greater knowledge about appropriate ways to influence the content of diet, the physical and social environment in which the malnourished live, and the distribution of food.

What Needs To Be Done?

INCREASING FOOD SUPPLY

Food production in the developing countries must increase at an unprecedented rate to the end of the century.

Eight food sources—rice, wheat, corn, sugar, cattle, sorghum, millet, and cassava—provide most of the nutrients for people in the developing countries. These eight food sources also are the major sources of income for people in those countries. They account for about three-fourths of the calories and two-thirds of the protein consumed, and in the case of the poorest populations may account for as much as 85 to 90 percent of calories and protein. Grains provide more than 60 percent of the calories consumed in the developing countries and perhaps 70 percent in the poorer countries, and they are the principal food commodity in world trade. Thus quantitative appraisals of the world food problem have concentrated primarily on grains. (See Table 1, Appendix A.)

Although grains are a useful basis for estimating approximate food balances, it is essential to recognize the importance of many other foods consumed in the developing countries. Potatoes, yams and sweet potatoes, beans and peas, nuts, fruits and vegetables, and animal products (including fish) are important sources of calories, protein, and other essential nutrients, and in many cases they are growing in importance as sources of farm income and foreign exchange.

Supply and Demand to Date in the Developing Countries

Between 1950 and 1975, food production in the developing countries as a whole (excluding China) expanded at the unprecedented rate of about 2.8 percent per year. The expansion was faster than that of the high-income countries, particularly between 1965 and 1975 when the results of agricultural research were applied increasingly to production (see Figure 3). However, since 1960 population and income growth in the developing countries have increased the demand for food by about 3.5 percent per year. Since production has not increased as rapidly, grain imports have filled much of the gap (see Table 1).

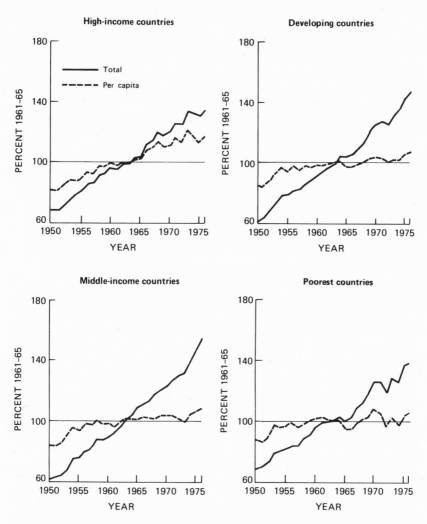

FIGURE 3   Food production indices: total and per capita, 1950–1976 (1961–65 = 100). From U.S. Department of Agriculture, Economic Research Service (1977).

TABLE 1   Average annual grain production, consumption, and imports for poorest and middle-income countries, and exports from principal sources (1,000 tons), 1961-63 to 1976

	1961–63	1964–66	1969–71	1973–75	1976
Poorest countries*					
Production	127,486	128,358	160,306	171,744	180,442
Consumption	133,569	140,947	165,630	181,652	188,212
Net imports	6,415	11,754	6,682	12,100	10,334
Gross imports	8,582	13,513	8,213	13,686	12,360
Middle-income countries**					
Production	99,653	113,110	129,772	143,145	167,240
Consumption	98,862	109,056	135,222	151,999	167,617
Net imports	451	–3,805	5,143	10,356	2,870
Gross imports	11,371	11,911	19,063	25,632	25,572
Exports from principal sources					
United States	36,889	44,314	39,692	74,499	76,724
Canada	12,692	14,804	15,293	15,099	16,730
Australia	6,754	7,617	10,767	11,026	12,410
Argentina	6,818	9,408	8,051	9,445	14,365
Thailand	2,273	2,755	3,433	3,812	3,550
European Community	7,630	11,453	17,791	25,708	13,207

*Poorest countries are those with per capita incomes of less than $200 in 1975. A list of these countries is included in Appendix A, Table 2.
**Middle-income countries are those with per capita incomes of over $200 in 1975. A list of these countries is included in Appendix A, Table 2.

SOURCE: U.S. Department of Agriculture, Economic Research Service (1977).

Despite the return of overall food production to the previous high growth trend of 2.8 percent, after the lull of 1972 to 1974, population growth has held average per capita increases in food production over the 1960 to 1975 period to about 0.3 percent per year. This leaves relatively little room to reduce malnutrition, particularly when the increased per capita consumption by the more affluent in these countries is taken into account. For the poorest group of developing countries, the average annual increase in food production has been only 2.3 percent over the past 15 years. Per capita consumption has not increased at all, and in Africa it has decreased by 10 percent.

Future Needs

The developing countries need to increase food production by about 3 to 4 percent per year to the end of the century. This estimate is based on:

- about 2.5 percent for annual population increases, if these stay at present levels;*
- about 1 percent for average annual increases in per capita food consumption, which seems a minimum goal given present levels of malnutrition, or more if declines in the rate of population growth permit;
- maintaining roughly the current proportion of their food supply that comes from net grain imports (about 15 percent of grain consumption in recent years for the importing countries) on the assumption that they probably cannot import more over long periods because of balance-of-payments problems.

The 3 to 4 percent estimate allows for considerable differences in these three factors among countries and over time; some countries may need to attain higher rates of growth of food production.

Expanded crop area or higher production per hectare per year are the only sources for the 3 to 4 percent crop production increases that are needed.

Annual increases in crop area probably will not exceed an average of 1 percent per year over the next 25 years, and may be appreciably less. Annual increases in crop area in the developing countries averaged 1.4 percent in the 1960s, declining over the decade. While costly programs are being planned or implemented to settle large new areas in Latin America and elsewhere, higher returns usually can be realized from investments on existing farmland. We assume that high costs and other typical difficulties will continue to slow development of new lands. *Thus adequate food supplies for the low-income areas of the world depend on substantial increases in production per hectare, averaging about 2.5 percent per year over the next 20 to 25 years.* Areas that are experiencing rapid population growth and lack land reserves may require increases in yields from 3 to 5 percent per year.

Prospects for Food Production in the Developing Countries

The average annual increase in crop yields in the developing countries was 1.9 percent during the 1960s. Achieving the needed increases in yield and output will not be easy. However, the 38 percent increase in the food production of the developing countries between 1965 and 1975 is encouraging, although expanding crop area may have played a greater role than it will in the future. Of the 71 countries on which we

* Assumptions about rates of population growth underlying our recommendation are discussed briefly in Appendix E.

have data for the 1965 to 1975 period (see Appendix A), 30 countries containing 1.3 billion people achieved or went beyond the estimated 3 to 4 percent rate of production increase needed for the future.

However, most of the poorest countries are only beginning to develop the capabilities needed to support a rising rate of productivity. They lack the capital, skills, and organization necessary for development. Because of their greater poverty and malnutrition, the poorest countries need proportionately larger annual increases in per capita food supply than the middle-income developing countries, and they can least afford continuing large-scale imports to supplement their own production.

Unprecedented rates of agricultural development are unlikely to occur without organizing special programs. These must be built around higher yielding farming systems, supported by adequate price incentives for greater production. Provisions must be made for adequate supplies of water, fertilizer, energy, and other inputs, and for marketing. Land tenure needs changing in many countries. Credit and other services must be provided. Large numbers of people must be trained and extension services strengthened. Research capabilities must be greatly strengthened. Price, trade, budget, and other policies must support an integrated development effort. Developing the capabilities to do all these things adequately is a formidable undertaking for the developing countries.

Implications for U.S. Production

The foregoing estimates of developing country requirements have important implications for the United States. The prospect that the developing countries will expand grain consumption and imports, parallel with their production increases, implies expanded exports for the United States. The expected growth of demand for U.S. food production both from U.S. sources and from other high-income countries must be added to this. We can, therefore, anticipate rising pressures on U.S. production costs and food prices unless research and development efforts succeed in reducing per unit costs of additional food production by increasing productivity. Productivity must continue to grow not only in the United States and other high-income countries but also to an equal or greater degree in the developing countries to counter rising costs of food production.

REDUCING POVERTY

Hunger and malnutrition cannot be addressed solely by food programs. The processes of social and economic development must be considered, including programs concerned with access to resources, distribution of income, control of parasitic and other infectious diseases, extension of health services, provision of safe water supplies, and literacy and general education.

In most countries, social, economic, and political measures not directly related to food are necessary to reduce malnutrition and improve health. National development programs should foster overall growth and improve incomes to reduce the extreme poverty that deprives people of adequate food. Direct food distribution can be used to supplement such programs.

Most developing countries are seeking accelerated growth of output and income. Many countries want to achieve a more equitable distribution of income. Given a developing country's commitment to these goals, success in reducing poverty heavily depends on rapidly expanding employment and labor productivity, and on a more plentiful food supply. Improving the productivity of small farms contributes to both of these objectives.

Maximum use of the available work force expands output and raises personal incomes, particularly at the lower end of the income scale. Expansion of the food supply allows the rural and urban poor to purchase food, their principal consumption item, at lower cost; this, combined with increased employment, raises their real incomes.

Expansion of national output complements expansion of food production and consumption. If the developing countries can maintain GNP increases near the level of about 6 percent achieved since 1960, the market demand for food will be adequate to absorb per capita supply increases of 1 to 2 percent.

Political support must be mobilized in support of the integrated expansion of output, employment, and food supply. This overall process would require:

– Changing national and international policies and institutions to improve income distribution and to implement effective development plans. Additional changes are required for improving health, education, shelter, credit, and other services that increase individual productivity and well-being and provide more income-generating opportunities. Better land tenure and improved distribution of water, grazing, and fishing rights also can be extremely important.
– Allowing scarce capital and capital goods to command prices covering full costs in order to encourage better use of available labor, increase of savings, and the channeling of savings toward the most productive investment uses. The composite effect generally is increased labor productivity and income.

– Developing domestic and export markets to permit rapid expansion of food production without sharp declines in price during periods of high production.

Direct food distribution programs can alleviate the more severe effects of poverty on nutrition in many countries. For example, supplemental feeding can be arranged for nutritionally vulnerable groups, such as pregnant and nursing mothers and preschool children, particularly in town or urban settings. Unemployed poor can be hired for rural public works and paid in food. Subsidies or government-guaranteed low prices for basic food requirements can be provided to low-income consumers through special retailers, food stamps, or other means. However, administrative, social, and political difficulties usually limit the extent to which such measures can reduce the large numbers of malnourished. Maldistribution of food can best be corrected over the longer term by providing poor people with the means and opportunities to produce or purchase more food.

STABILIZING FOOD SUPPLY

Local, national, and international measures are needed to prevent sudden sharp drops in food supplies and to prevent severe market gluts that discourage production.

One need is to focus on problems occurring at the farm level. Improved technology can reduce losses of crops and livestock caused by weather and pests. Production research must emphasize both increasing and stabilizing yields.

Farmers would benefit substantially from improved weather prediction. Weather and climate modification is a more uncertain and long-term prospect calling for full exploration.

Research also can identify governmental options for reducing instability in food supplies and prices that result from inappropriate policies. For example, governments frequently do not allow the price shifts needed to induce changes in consumption or production, which would moderate conditions of food shortage or surplus. Or, they may remove food supplies from national and international markets and thereby increase instability in those markets.

One of the most effective remedies for removing cycles of glut and shortage continues to be Joseph's prescription for the Pharaoh—increased food reserves coupled with effective stockpile management. Better food preservation and storage methods are needed in the developing countries both at the farm level and beyond. These should be supplemented by improved international storage and emergency transfer arrangements.

The United States and other high-income countries could underwrite agreements that would ensure participating nations against temporary serious shortfalls in food production. Such programs should be carefully designed to avoid discouraging local production or the development of local grain reserves.

It is important that action be taken to reduce cycles of glut and shortage and also that they not be allowed to distort perspectives on the more serious longer-term problem. The essential course of action to solve the basic food shortage problem is a long, steady effort to raise the productivity of agricultural resources in order at least to double the production of food by the end of the century and provide further increases thereafter. A few consecutive years of good harvest should not divert us from this purpose.

IMPROVING FOOD AND NUTRITION POLICY

A few poor countries have achieved levels of life expectancy, infant mortality, and death rates and birth rates usually achieved only in societies with much higher incomes. Sri Lanka and the Indian state of Kerala, while their per capita incomes were less than $150, and South Korea, Taiwan, and, probably, China, while their per capita incomes were still less than $300, are five such cases. If other low-income countries had similar death and birth rates, the number of deaths each year would decrease by more than 10 million and the number of births would be reduced far more.

These heartening results seem to be associated with a wide range of food transfer, education, health delivery, land tenure, and other labor-intensive rural programs, but far too little is known about specific relationships and the different circumstances involved. This knowledge is essential as a basis for action, and would inform decision makers about the nutritional gains that can be achieved, and about the outcomes of inaction.

Governments of developing countries that are trying to establish rational nutrition policies and programs need encouragement and support. The United States also lacks and needs adequate research and policy mechanisms in this field. Collaboration and exchanges of information between the developing countries and the United States are essential to build nutrition policy research capabilities on both sides.

POPULATION

In the long run, no action is more important for improving the world food and nutrition situation than reducing the high birth rates that still prevail in much of the world.

Significant gains in nutrition in the low-income countries may have the short-run effect of increasing population growth rates by decreasing mortality rates before birth rates decline. However, there is increasing evidence for the hypothesis that the kinds of social and economic changes required for major increases in food production and better health also are conducive to later marriage, lower fertility, and successful policies to reduce birth rates. The developing countries must substantially increase food production both to provide for the short-run population increase that is inevitable and, as part of integrated development, to induce socioeconomic changes that will result in a rapid, sustained reduction in fertility. Recommending research on specific population interventions is beyond our mandate. However, U.S. research capabilities are contributing far less than they could to expanding the options for achieving the population changes so urgently required in many countries.

• *We strongly recommend that the U.S. government sponsor a study to assess how U.S. research capabilities can be best applied to help countries that desire effective means of reducing birth rates.*

The study should cover biological, socioeconomic, policy, and organizational factors. It should assess current demographic status and trends worldwide, and should recommend measures to strengthen the usefulness of U.S. research resources for the world population situation.

The Role of Research

The role of research is to broaden the range of choices available to all who influence world food supply and nutrition: farmers, consumers, agribusiness managers, health service personnel, government officials, and politicians. Sustaining a flow of improved choices to these decision makers is crucial if world hunger and malnutrition are to be reduced by the end of the century. In stressing this, we do not wish to promote the notion that research and development will solve world food problems, only that it is an essential part of the solution. Many other factors must be considered in guiding research into productive paths and in applying the improved options that research makes possible. These options must, of course, fit well into particular development contexts. Moreover, even when they do fit well, difficult and time-consuming adjustment processes may be required for existing systems to accommodate new ways of doing things. Many of these complicating factors are themselves in need of research that can identify better ways of coping with them. Research is needed to improve the results that are attainable with limited resources, recognizing the important role that adequate resources and policy play in development.

THE RESEARCH SPECTRUM

The improvement of food systems, from production through consumption, requires a continuum starting with adapting existing technologies and resources to local needs, moving to improving technologies within the limits of available scientific knowledge, and ending with a search for new scientific discoveries that extend the biological, physical, and social limits of knowledge. Fundamental work with large potential to improve technology should be pursued now because results typically will not affect food supplies for 10 or 20 years.

Research is particularly important to improve development policies and organizations in order to assure that technologies affecting food production and consumption are appropriate to the social and economic goals and environments of each country. The kinds of technologies used in the developing countries influence the relative shares of national income received by the poor and hence the degrees of poverty and malnutrition. This consideration underlies our selection of research and development priorities. We stress biological innovations, farming systems, and risk-reducing technologies that will most benefit the lowest-income farmers and farm laborers. We also emphasize research that concentrates on those who are malnourished; that illuminates the socioeconomic effects of organizational, policy, and technology choices; and that helps to reconcile food needs with requirements for conserving and enhancing the earth's natural resources.

THE IMPORTANCE OF MORE BASIC RESEARCH

Large-scale improvements in technology are needed to achieve long-term goals such as: a sustained 3 to 4 percent annual growth rate of developing country food production; a reduced dependence worldwide on chemical and other energy-intensive production inputs; and a major improvement in the nutritional status of the world population. Applied research to provide technologies and policies needed to advance toward such goals is severely constrained by a lack of scientific knowledge about biological and behavioral factors.

We need to know more about the interactions within and between the elements of the natural and social systems relating to our food supply (e.g., plants and animals and their organs, cells, and smaller components; disease agents; soils; atmosphere; the human body; and individual, family, and community behavior mechanisms) and about the cause-and-effect relationships underlying what is happening. With such knowledge, researchers can improve techniques for changing existing relationships among these elements. It also can provide the basis for larger-scale and more rapid improvements in the performance characteristics of plants and animals, for improving the nutritional effects of food, and for enhancing the effectiveness of organizations and policies governing food systems.

It is essential to pursue basic research that can be useful in removing impediments to *worldwide* technological gains, and to accelerate gains in fundamental knowledge that bear upon specific applied research problems. For example, basic genetic research may provide plants and microorganisms with the capacity to fix nitrogen. Applied research would then make it possible to introduce this yield-determining characteristic into crops grown around the world.

GAINS FROM RESEARCH

Analyses of investments in agricultural research generally indicate that returns have been several times those usually realized by other types of industrial or developmental investment. Evenson's study (1975) of average benefits from wheat and rice research in some two dozen countries estimates that, for the period 1948 to 1971, each dollar of basic agricultural research generated, after 8 to 10 years, an annual benefit of about $80 in developing countries and $31 in high-income countries. The equivalent estimates for applied or developmental agricultural research were about $60 and $7. These estimates must be interpreted with caution, but they are evidence that the annual returns from investment in research on food production may be as much as 40 to 60 percent in the developing countries.

Studies indicate that a major factor in the higher rate of return from research investment in the developing countries is the large potential for using and adapting knowledge from research performed elsewhere. Studies also indicate that a developing country needs a significant research capacity of its own to profit from outside research.

The strength of exchanges between national research and outside research, and between farmers and researchers, is a key determinant of the return from national research.

Basic research can open up unexpected applications of great value, apart from its value in attacking preidentified bottlenecks to progress in applied research. For example, the possibilities of selecting out and recombining particular genetic components of diverse organisms (recombinant DNA), originally discovered by biomedical research, could mean increasing agricultural yields. Work by a USDA scientist on the structure of the RNA molecule is of profound value in the design of fertilizers for plant use, among other important practical applications.

Basic bacteriological studies led to using urea and other nonprotein nitrogens as feed supplements for ruminants, thereby substantially reducing the cost of beef. These supplements currently substitute for some of the protein in ruminant rations, and thus free natural proteins, such as soybean meal, for human consumption. Basic research on antibiotics has been applied to animals in the United States, with a reported annual savings of approximately $1 billion. Such examples are numerous.

The Role of the United States

Clearly, each country must chart its own course of development and select the technological components it regards as appropriate. Each country is responsible for solving its own problems of malnutrition and poverty. We do not assume superior wisdom concerning these matters on the part of this Committee or on the part of other U.S. groups. We assume only a U.S. capability and willingness to work and collaborate on research problems where U.S. participation is welcomed.

The United States, along with other high-income nations, can help solve food problems by measures that are beyond the scope of this study, for example, by providing capital assistance, by cooperating in the formulation of development plans, and by working for more effective international policies on trade and on management of cereal reserves. We believe that larger U.S. involvement in these activities is desirable.

Here, we are concerned with research on food and nutrition, and we believe the United States should contribute far more to world needs in this area. The United States has extensive experience in and facilities for planning, organizing, and conducting research and for educating scientific personnel. One recent estimate puts the U.S. expenditure for publicly supported agricultural research at almost a third of the world total.

The United States can contribute by helping to build research capabilities in the developing countries and by orienting U.S. research activities more to global concerns about hunger and malnutrition.

THE U.S. RESEARCH ROLE

The United States can assist developing countries in building their food and nutrition research capabilities by helping them to establish and operate research institutions, and by helping to train scientists and other research workers. Research capabilities also can be strengthened on both sides if U.S. and developing country research organizations collaborate on joint research projects, exchanges of research information and materials, exchanges of scientists and students, technical conferences, and advisory services.

Research that shapes and fits available technologies to local circumstances is indispensable for using improved technology. This research must be performed locally. Often technology is not applied more widely in developing countries because localities are unable to adapt it to their particular circumstances. Therefore it is natural that research institutions in the developing countries place high priority on building capabilities for adaptive research that can bring relatively quick production results. At the same time, the developing countries should build up their own basic research skills. Some have made substantial progress in this regard.

Our choices of priorities for additional U.S. research have been made in the context of world research. The United States is only one of many possible sources of additional support for work on world food problems. Other high-income countries, many international organizations and, most important of all, the developing countries are making increased efforts. Thus the U.S. research community should emphasize those activities that it can do best, while recognizing the need to work with research organizations outside the United States. Clearly, research that benefits the United States domestically has the best prospect of sustaining more and higher quality U.S. support over the long term.

U.S. and developing country interests are best served if U.S. research relevant to both concentrates on work that requires the highly trained scientists and complex research facilities abundant in the United States, and that generates results that are widely transferable to the developing countries for incorporation into further research and development there. Three categories of research fit these criteria well:

(1) basic research; (2) comparative analysis of the experiences of different countries with similar technical, social, or policy innovations; and (3) development of analytical and research methodologies.

Obtaining significant results from the last two types of research, involving predominantly social science analysis, is difficult. All countries are short of good research results and capabilities in this field. But the United States is relatively well supplied with the requisite tools: working experience in countries around the world, highly trained social science analysts, and rapid access to worldwide data. We should expand this important work.

In emphasizing fundamental biological research and the need to integrate social science research into food and nutrition research and development programs, we do not want to appear to understate the importance of conventional applied agricultural research. The latter provides the means to translate knowledge from fundamental biological and socioeconomic research into improved technology that can be used by farmers. Thus it is essential to strengthen conventional research in such areas as plant and animal breeding, soil and water management, cultivation practices, mechanization, animal feeding and health, environmental stresses and stability of yields, and improvement of capital inputs.

BUILDING RESEARCH COOPERATION

The effect of U.S. research on world food problems depends on the effectiveness of U.S. working relationships with national and international research and development organizations in the developing countries. Better collaboration also is needed among the disparate U.S. research communities. There is very little working contact between those engaged in fundamental research in the biological sciences and those involved in technological research on food and nutrition problems.

The contrast between agriculture and medicine is instructive. In the case of medicine, fundamental research in the biological sciences is closely linked to applied medical research through large-scale funding by the National Institutes of Health and by major medical schools. This has not been done to nearly the same extent in agriculture. Links between nutrition or food science departments and strong biological research units also are too limited. The result is that most of the workers in fundamental biological research in the United States have gravitated to the biomedical side. More of them should be attracted into the food area.

BENEFITS OF RESEARCH COLLABORATION

The United States and developing countries have common interests in research collaboration that would provide the following benefits:

- Reduced production costs that increase the profitability of farming; stimulate food output, development, and reciprocal trade; permit more stable food prices; and help control inflationary pressures.
- Reduced year-to-year fluctuations in world supplies of grains and other major foods, which are accompanied by sharp price fluctuations that cause economic difficulties for U.S. and developing country farmers and consumers.
- Reduced environmental pollution and consumption of energy and scarce minerals.
- Increased knowledge about the complex interrelationships among diet, health, life-style, and factors in the physical and socioeconomic environments.

The United States will benefit from an expanded flow of technical findings from production research in the developing countries. Germ plasm developed through programs in the developing countries has improved the yields and stress resistances of U.S. crops and will be increasingly important in pest resistance. Some examples of technical findings from the developing countries of benefit to the United States are:

- Virus-resistant Pangola grass from South America has restored large beef pastures in the Southeast.
- Nigerian beans of high nutritional quality have been adapted by Wisconsin researchers.
- Wong barley from China established barley as an important crop on the Eastern Seaboard.
- The high yielding Hudson potato, incorporating Andean genes, has been widely used.
- Lentil varieties from Turkey have given the first successful winter production of lentils and show high promise in the Pacific Northwest.
- One wheat variety collected in Turkey is estimated to have benefited the United States by $50 million annually.
- Two soybean varieties introduced from Nanking, China, have given impetus to large-scale soybean production in the southern United States.
- Oat varieties from Israel now give the best protection possible in the United States from crown rust infestation.

– International wheat research centers also have furnished the United
States with such high yielding varieties as the "lancota" variety, re-
leased jointly in 1975 by USDA and university scientists in Nebraska,
Kansas, South Dakota, and Texas. Similarly, crossbreeding of traditional English breeds with foreign beef cattle such as Brahma and
Charolais types has improved the disease and parasite resistance of
animals in the South and Southwest.

Research and development on nutrition problems in the developing
countries could improve the health and well-being of all peoples. The
United States is already applying at home knowledge gained from research and development collaboration on food fortification in the developing countries. Similarly, studies of patterns of disease in the
developing countries are contributing to U.S. research that is exploring
possible links between diets and cancer, coronary heart disease, and
other illnesses that afflict Americans. Large savings in health service
costs may be realized.

Two additional benefits from international research collaboration
deserve emphasis. First, expanding food production by raising productivity is perhaps the most effective way to moderate the disruptive
struggles between producers and consumers over food prices. This
struggle within and between countries is a major source of domestic
and international discord. With growth in productivity, producers can
receive lower prices up to a point and still gain income. An important
role for policy research is to find ways to assure that rising yields benefit
both producers and consumers and to moderate short-term costs of
technological change for groups that might be harmed.

Second, the mutual gains in knowledge from international collaboration on research and development are important. This collaboration
provides the developing countries access to the world's knowledge base,
which is crucial to their development efforts. It gives the United States
an opportunity to enhance its understanding of other peoples, particularly those who live in developing countries. Direct experience in problem solving in foreign environments is a good way to strengthen the U.S.
knowledge base. Participants from universities and other organizations
gain understanding needed to train people in all fields who must relate
increasingly to the world around us.

Action Proposed

In light of the foregoing assessment, we recommend in the following
chapters U.S. actions that would expand and strengthen our research

and development contribution to solving world food and nutrition problems.

First, we recommend research that could improve food and nutrition policies, increase food availability, reduce poverty, and stabilize food supplies.

Second, we recommend actions to help mobilize and organize research and development resources in the United States and worldwide.

Third, we recommend a mechanism to better integrate U.S. government actions that affect food and nutrition throughout the world.

The size of the research effort that we recommend for the United States is moderate and feasible. The additional cost would average about $210 to $230 million per year over the first four years of the program. This is approximately 1 percent of the federal research and development budget and 10 percent of the estimated total food and nutrition research done in the United States.

An Opportunity

The world's food problems present a challenge to U.S. research capabilities. This challenge, although difficult and urgent, is attended by many reasons for optimism.

Our most important reason for optimism is the increasing ability of many developing countries to address their own food problems. While progress over the past decade has been uneven and many difficulties remain, the present situation includes:

- larger numbers of trained, experienced technical and managerial people in the institutions serving agriculture and marketing;
- clearer perceptions on the part of policymakers and officials about what is needed to improve food systems and accelerate the pace of development;
- greater availability of the tools of production—fertilizers, water, farm capital, and supporting services, including research;
- a labor supply that facilitates the use of intensive farming practices that can result in high yields per hectare with relatively small capital inputs;
- availability of a wide array of external assistance;
- greater agreement among the nations and organizations of the world about the nature of the problems.

The unique potential and problems of tropical agriculture are beginning to be recognized. Wide variations in climate and soils in tropical regions require many different kinds of technology. Efforts to control soil, disease, pest, and other problems of tropical agriculture, and efforts to identify more productive farming systems for different tropical areas are still in their early stages. Year-round or relatively long annual growing seasons are common. The potential for increasing food production appears to be great, but there must be full recognition of the importance of avoiding serious ecological damage.

The potential for improving yields in the developing countries is very large, as indicated by the disparities in yields of major food crops and animal products among different countries and different producers. For example, FAO data on rice yields for 1975 show a few countries in the 5 to 6 tons per hectare* range, but three-fourths of the 115 countries included had average yields under 3 tons, and over half were under 2 tons. Similar data for maize yields show 82 countries producing under 1.5 tons per hectare in contrast to average yields of 5.4 tons in the United States. Average dry bean yields in the Far East are about one-fourth of yields in the Near East. Many factors account for such differences, but adaptive research to fit known technology to local circumstances, together with adequate policy support and organizational services, could greatly reduce them.

There are large reserve assets in the developing countries that can be applied over the long run to increase world food production, and research can help make them more useful. These assets include large areas of land suitable for farming; grossly underutilized water resources; many sources of fertilizer and animal feed, including organic wastes, that we can learn to use more efficiently; food currently lost during or after production; and large quantities of waste products from grains, oilseeds, fish, and animals that are now thrown away or used for nonfood purposes.

Many developing countries have made important progress in addressing poverty and population growth, two factors that influence malnutrition. We have noted the rapid advances of national output and income since 1960. While the absolute numbers of those malnourished and living in absolute poverty have increased, the proportion of their populations in these conditions has declined. Recently, balance-of-payments problems, stemming primarily from rising petroleum prices, have disrupted economic progress for many of the poorest countries. However, most developing country governments are pursuing rapid development nevertheless. The meeting of basic human needs is gaining support as an important goal for development although there has been little progress in improving the distribution of money income. For example, there are increasing efforts to reach larger numbers of people

---

* Metric measures are used throughout this report.

with public health and other services aimed at reducing the effect of poverty on nutrition. Many countries have experienced substantial drops in birth rates since 1965, notably in Asia.

Capitalizing on these promising elements will not be easy. In many cases, it will require structural reforms that are politically difficult, large outlays of capital, and tenacious efforts. Because of such difficulties, progress could be slow.

On the other hand, if there is the political will in this country and abroad to capitalize on these elements, it should be possible to overcome the worst aspects of widespread hunger and malnutrition within one generation. By the end of the century, food production could be doubled in the developing countries. In the high-income countries, grain production could be increased by more than the total grain production of the United States today, even while maintaining reasonable production costs despite the rising costs of energy, water, and other requirements. We find these prospects exciting and worthy of strong national and international efforts, and we believe that a latent political will now exists in numerous countries which could be mobilized in a mutually supporting fashion to commence and support such efforts.

The 1974 World Food Conference, from which this study resulted, was a major first step in mobilizing the world community to address the problems of increasing world food production and reducing hunger and malnutrition. Continuous, if slow, progress has been made in following up on some of the conference's principal resolutions, including the establishment of a World Food Council and of an International Fund for Agricultural Development. In mid-1976, the World Employment Conference focused attention on the potential for more effectively addressing basic human needs, and on the possibilities, through cooperative efforts, for removing hunger and malnutrition as a major scourge by the end of this century. The U.S. government has prescribed new directions for U.S. development assistance that recognize that good nutrition and productive employment are essential to human well-being. And late in 1976, both the U.S. Senate and U.S. House of Representatives passed essentially similar resolutions enunciating a "right" to food. We find these steps encouraging.

In his statement to the citizens of the world broadcast on Inauguration Day, President Carter said that the United States will cooperate with other peoples in shaping a world order that is more responsive to human aspirations, including cooperation in fulfilling the basic human right to be free of poverty and hunger. He also said that the United States will take the lead in furthering such cooperation. The recommendations of this study identify practical ways in which the United States can pursue this resolve.

2 High Priority Research

Chapter 2 presents major research areas and promising approaches for achieving them. In keeping with the President's request, the selection of research areas was based on their prospective effects on world hunger over the next few decades. Details of proposed research are given in the *Supporting Papers*.

We identify research areas that need larger U.S. research expenditures. Some food and nutrition research that is important may be adequately funded already. We are not attempting to recommend the full set of priorities for U.S. research in this field. Many types of research are under way in U.S. facilities for good reasons unrelated to this study.

How Priorities Were Established

To establish a set of research areas which should have priority, 12 interdisciplinary study teams of experts were assembled (see Table 2) and each team was asked to identify outstanding areas of research and development required to help meet world food and nutrition needs. Three questions posed by the Steering Committee guided the selection of priorities:

— What advances in knowledge will specific areas of research produce, and what is the scientific or technological significance of these advances?

— If the research produces results, what effect would they likely have

TABLE 2   Study teams, World Food and Nutrition Study

Study Team	Title	
1	Crop Productivity	
	Subgroup A	Pest Control
2	Animal Productivity	
	Subgroup A	Animal Health
3	Aquatic Food Sources	
4	Resources for Agriculture	
	Subgroup A	Farming Systems
	B	Land and Water
	C	Fertilizers
	D	Energy and Equipment
5	Weather and Climate	
6	Food Availability to Consumers	
	Subgroup A	Food Losses
	B	Food Processing and Preservation
	C	Food Marketing and Distribution
7	Rural Institutions, Policies, and Social Science Research	
	Subgroup A	Policies and Program Planning
	B	Research, Education and Training, and Extension
	C	Finance, Input Supplies, and Farmers' Organizations
8	Information Systems	
9	Nutrition	
10	Interdependencies	
	Subgroup A	Population and Health
	B	Energy, Resources, and Environment
	C	International Trade Policy and Comity Between Nations
	D	National Development Policies
11	New Approaches to Increasing Food Supplies	
12	New Approaches to the Alleviation of Hunger	
13	Research Priority Assessment	
14	Agricultural Research Organization	
	Subgroup A	Research Organization in the United States
	B	Global Agricultural Research Organization
	C	Development of Research Personnel

on reducing global hunger and malnutrition over the next several decades?

– What supportive action will be required to conduct research for the accelerated activity recommended (e.g., more resources, policy changes, organizational changes)?

The study teams began with assessments of research priorities already made by U.S. and international agencies. In light of their own experience and after consulting hundreds of other experts, they produced a list of over 100 priority research areas. This list was then analyzed by Study Team 13, composed of 19 experts of broad background and experience in food and nutrition. Study Team 13 ranked the research areas according to near-term effects (less than 15 years) and longer term effects (beyond 15 years). (The ranking process is explained in more detail in Appendix B.) Final adjustments in priorities were made by the Steering Committee.

The results of this selection process are presented as 22 priority research areas in four categories: nutrition, food production, food marketing, and policies and organizations. No rankings are made among the 22 areas; they constitute the minimum of a highly selected list of promising areas of research requiring support. Research in each priority area addresses a broad research goal. Within each area we recommend particular lines of research that we believe to be the most promising for additional U.S. support.

• *We recommend that U.S. research support be increased for the lines of research identified within these 22 research areas:*

- Nutrition–Performance Relations
- Role of Dietary Components
- Policies Affecting Nutrition
- Nutrition Intervention Programs
- Plant Breeding and Genetic Manipulation
- Biological Nitrogen Fixation
- Photosynthesis
- Resistance to Environmental Stresses
- Pest Management
- Weather and Climate
- Management of Tropical Soils
- Irrigation and Water Management
- Fertilizer Sources
- Ruminant Livestock

- Aquatic Food Sources
- Farm Production Systems
- Postharvest Losses
- Market Expansion
- National Food Policies and Organizations
- Trade Policy
- Food Reserves
- Information Systems

The recommended areas include both basic and applied research. All of the research is mission-oriented; that is, each priority line of research was selected because of a significant probability that, if successful, it would contribute to the improvement of the world food and nutrition situation. Research, of course, must be translated into effectively operating technologies and programs.

BALANCING LONG-TERM AND SHORT-TERM RESEARCH

Some recommended research areas could produce results in the developing countries and in the United States within 5 to 15 years. Others will produce results only over the longer term. This study identifies research areas that attempt to balance the need for long-term research that has major payoffs with the need for short-term research that has smaller but more immediate returns.

Nitrogen research presents an example of the choices that face the government. The amount of nitrogen available to food plants is a fundamental limitation to expanding food production worldwide. There are many ways to reduce this limitation. Applying more of the available nitrogen fertilizers will produce the most immediate returns on investment. Improving fertilizers and existing symbiotic interactions between legumes and nitrogen-fixing bacteria is expected to produce results in both the near and distant future. Research on new forms of biological nitrogen fixation and on organic recycling of nitrogen will require more time before results can be expected.

The strategic question is how best to allocate resources. This decision must take into account probable improvements in yield from existing technology, likely trends in food supply and demand, prospects for significant new research results at different levels of effort, and the probable length of time required for research to produce results. Socioeconomic effects also must be weighed.

For example, research to alter biological processes so that crops could fix more nitrogen could mean less dependence on chemical fertilizers: this could reduce food production costs, pollution, and the drain on stocks of petroleum and natural gas, and would be of particular benefit to small farmers in the developing countries. These prospects for such dramatic payoffs lead us to believe that there is an urgent need to accelerate research on biological nitrogen fixation in crops. Similarly, with the same urgency research should be accelerated on photosynthesis and new techniques for genetic manipulation, and on some longer term elements of research in other priority areas described below.

We conclude that the United States has not given adequate attention to the long lead time required in bringing basic research to application.

WHERE IS THE RESEARCH SUPPORT NEEDED?

Table 3 lists the research goal and priority lines of research in each of the 22 priority areas. It also includes anticipated effects of the research and suggests possible sources of federal financing.

The proportion of U.S.-financed research that should be done in the United States and the proportion that should be done in the developing countries vary among the types of research. In Chapter 1, we suggest that the United States should support research in both places for most research recommended and should foster collaboration between work in this country and that being undertaken in other high-income countries.

Our priorities give special weight to research for which large parts of the U.S.-financed work can be done in the United States. Such research can produce major benefits both here and in the developing countries. Such research is comprised of the more basic types of research, comparative analyses of worldwide experience, and methodological studies. Such an orientation increases the scope for strong and enduring U.S. research support on problems that are important for developing countries. Nevertheless, our organizational recommendations stress expanding U.S. support for building research capabilities in developing countries, including the provision of research funds that each country can apply to its own priorities.

Nutrition

Nutrition is fundamental to human life, performance, and well-being. Levels of nutritional well-being both influence and reflect social and economic development in every country. This report discusses priorities for various parts of the food system, from primary production to final

TABLE 3 Recommended research priorities

Priority area	Nature of research effort	Major effects	Sources of support
I. Nutrition			
Nutrition-performance relations	Determine damage caused by various kinds and levels of malnutrition: effects of diet patterns on levels of human functioning	Nutritional improvement in short run; in long run dietary changes may benefit health and life expectancy of large population segments in United States; in developing countries nutritional interventions likely to be more effective for human health than comparable investments in medical care	NIH, NSF, USDA, AID
Role of dietary components	Determine specific foods that best meet nutritional needs under differing circumstances: effects of individual nutrient levels, as consumed, on nutritional status		
Policies affecting nutrition	Improve effects of full range of government policies: effects on nutrition of policies and practices usually formulated with no consideration of possible nutritional consequences		
Nutrition intervention programs	Improve effects of direct intervention programs: evaluate effectiveness of alternative programs in reaching nutritional goals		
II. Food production			
Plant breeding and genetic manipulation	Strengthen tools of genetic manipulation: plant breeding, and "classical" genetics; cell biology; genetic stocks	Worldwide potential is immense; production increases from most lines of research expected in 10 to 20 years; instrumental for progress in other priority areas	USDA, NSF, AID
Biological nitrogen fixation	Increase biological nitrogen fixation associated with major crops: improve recognized symbiotic associations; attempt to establish N_2-fixing associations with grains and other nonlegumes; transfer fixation capability from bacteria to plants	Large potential worldwide; results within 10 to 15 years for legumes and 15 to 25 years for nonlegumes	USDA, NSF, AID, EPA

Photosynthesis	Increase amount of photosynthesis in major crops: reducing photorespiration and dark respiration; transferring traits from photosynthetically efficient plants	Higher yields of food plants particularly in the tropics; substantial increases in potential yields after 15 years or more	USDA, NSF
Resistance to environmental stresses	Improve resistance of major crops to drought, temperature extremes, deficiencies of acid soils, salinity: rapid screening techniques; tolerance of acid soils; shorter season crops; larger root systems; better use of soil fungi; salinity resistance; farming systems	Larger and more stable crop yields in 10 to 15 years, more efficient use of inputs, possible to grow crops in new locations	USDA, NSF, AID
Pest management	Reduce preharvest losses due to pests: integrated pest management; specific control mechanisms	Can eliminate large and pervasive losses due to pests, in short run by adapting known technology, in long run by biological control techniques	USDA, NSF, AID, EPA
Weather and climate	Improve techniques for predicting weather and climate and using information to assist adaptation by farmers: reduce weather damage to food production	Substantial analytical improvement in short run; can have payoffs many times the cost	NOAA, USDA, NASA, NSF
Management of tropical soils	Improve management of tropical soils to increase crop productivity: soil classification; land clearing methods; correcting soil deficiencies; maintaining desired soil characteristics; suitable cropping systems and technologies	Annual crop production in humid lands can be 150 to 200 percent of temperate zone production per hectare	USDA, AID
Irrigation and water management	Improve management of water supplies: adjustments in farming systems and management of water movement for optimal supply to crops; adapting farming operations to water availability	May double crop yields in some areas, and make capital investments more effective	USDA, AID

TABLE 3 (Continued)

Priority area	Nature of research effort	Major effects	Sources of support
Fertilizer sources	Improve cost/return ratios of chemical fertilizers: new methods of producing nitrogen and phosphorus fertilizer; new fertilizers tailored to tropical conditions	Advances in short and long run; new ways of producing nitrogen fertilizer will reduce energy consumption; new and more efficient fertilizers could have major effects on tropical food production	AID, TVA, USDA, ERDA
Ruminant livestock	Increase product yields from ruminant livestock, particularly in the tropics: forages; priority animal diseases; genetics and reproduction	Forage and disease research will open up new areas and will improve productivity and eliminate heavy economic losses	USDA, AID, NSF
Aquatic food sources	Increase contribution of aquatic resources to world food supply: waste reduction and upgrading product through processing; aquaculture research in both breeding and seed supply and polyculture management	Could double fish protein consumed by humans without increasing world catch; could raise potential aquaculture yields fivefold	AID, DOI, DOC, NSF, USDA
Farm production systems	Improve production systems, particularly for small farms in developing countries: methodology for identifying appropriate farming system; multiple cropping; soil and water management; equipment-labor relationships	Realize potential for two to four times present production in humid tropics; more modest increases in semiarid tropics	AID, USDA, EPA, ERDA
III. *Food marketing* Postharvest losses	Reduce postharvest losses: nature and magnitude of losses; pest control after harvest; food preservation for humid and arid tropics	Substantial reduction in losses that now range 15 to 50 percent of production; encouragement of beneficial changes in cropping patterns	AID, NSF, USDA, DOD

Market expansion	Extend market scope for consumers and farmers in developing countries: enhancing purchasing power; transportation; marketing institutions; managing marketing flows of major commodities	Stimulate production and consumption and cut food losses: effects in 5 to 10 years	AID, USDA
IV. *Policies and organizations*			
National food policies and organizations	Improve policies and organizations affecting food production, distribution, and nutrition in developing countries: human performance in food systems; comparative studies to identify transferable improvement factors (decentralization, local participation, staff development); interactions of income distribution with food production and nutrition; methodology of sector analysis	Early results in improving effectiveness of policies and organizations relating to food systems and orienting selection and implementation of other biological and physical research; give farmers incentives for production and provide prices that will give more effective distribution	AID, NSF, USDA
Trade policy	Improve effects of trade policy on food production and nutrition: studies on effects of trade liberalization; consequences of international management of trade; optimum trading patterns	Early effects on orientating country food policies for balance between own production and reliance on trade; improve diets, incomes, and national economic performance	USDA, AID, State, DOC
Food reserves	Improve role of reserves in relation to other measures for stabilizing food supplies: improving developing country food reserve practices; identifying improved mixes of reserves and other measures to stabilize food supply	Relieve hunger and malnutrition due to production instability	USDA, AID
Information systems	Improve flows of information in support of decision making on food and nutrition: producer information needs to use better technology; crop monitoring systems; international data bases on land uses and malnutrition; information systems design	Large gains, especially in developing countries, from fewer wrong decisions and fuller use of available improved technologies	USDA, NASA, DOD, NOAA, AID

consumption, but all priorities are based on the goal of adequate nutrition for all segments of the world population.

Presently, nutritional deprivation is doing immense damage to human lives and societies throughout the world. For a nation, widespread malnutrition can mean impaired physical and mental growth and development of its children, reduced working capacity and income of its adults, increased costs from disease and health care, and high death rates. The intangible costs of reduced human vitality may be even greater.

Unfortunately, the national and international policies and activities that affect the nutritional status of world populations are seldom examined systematically to identify their effects on nutrition. Even programs designed to improve nutrition are rarely evaluated for their effectiveness. Research is needed not only on the extent and functional significance of malnutrition but also on the merit of present and future policies affecting food systems. Research in these areas could prevent a significant proportion of the disease presently attributed to malnutrition and its associated cost, and could improve the quality of human life and performance.

Much information already exists on the occurrence and importance of malnutrition in most countries, but far too little is known about the many factors that contribute to its cause. There is also not enough information on the nutritional requirements of different population groups, especially where poverty is prevalent. Little information is available on the relative costs and benefits of different national policies directed toward nutrition and of the effectiveness of international, bilateral, and nongovernmental efforts to assist nutrition programs. Moreover, social factors affect food distribution and nutritional status within the family, and these factors cannot be determined from knowledge of community food supplies alone or even of overall family consumption. Under these circumstances, decision makers frequently lack a firm basis for judging the effects of their actions and therefore have little incentive to give nutrition programs a high priority.

The research recommended in this section is specifically designed to prevent malnutrition by providing information for effective action. The types of knowledge being sought and their application are highly interdependent, and all merit high priority.

NUTRITION–PERFORMANCE RELATIONSHIPS

In order to survive, individuals who have low calorie intakes must reduce their physical activity. The discrepancy between estimated normal requirements and actual dietary intakes observed for the populations of most developing countries suggests that such reduced activity is widespread. However, neither the economic and social consequences of these low intakes of dietary energy nor the benefits of increasing them have been studied sufficiently. Similarly, iron deficiency anemia, which lowers performance and resistance to infection, is widespread. Information on the significance of this problem for specific countries is almost nonexistent. Protein–calorie deficiency is responsible for the poor growth of children in the developing countries. It impairs their performance on tests of learning and behavior and reduces their resistance to infection. However, the relative requirements for protein and calories and the effects of minimal deficiencies of each are highly controversial, largely because the requisite information is lacking. This is true for deficiencies of most other nutrients as well.

Types of Research

For the individual and for society, there is a need to determine the consequences of low levels of nutrition on work performance, frequency and severity of infection, physical and mental growth and development, school and job performance, pregnancy and lactation, and fertility and family planning. Research should emphasize how diets affect childbearing and childrearing functions. Information is needed on the extent to which the nutritional status of mothers affects the three variables that determine the biological potential for population growth: span of reproductive years, pace at which successive pregnancies occur, and rate of child survival. To decide which nutritional problems should receive priority and how resources may best be allocated among various target groups, it is essential to know the relative seriousness of different states of nutrition and the degree of benefit that can be derived from specific increments of nutritional improvement.

ROLE OF DIETARY COMPONENTS

Knowledge of requirements for particular nutrients is surprisingly fragmentary, even for the healthy populations of the high-income countries. Little specific information is known about the environmental circumstances and diets of those living in the developing countries. It is known that nutritional requirements are affected by the prevalence of acute and chronic infections, and that some nutrients are lacking in bulky, predominantly vegetable, diets. Knowledge about the extent to which specific foods and diets meet nutritional needs can guide decision makers who influence nutritional goals for agriculture, government support policies, food quality and safety, food distribution and marketing practices, supplementary feeding programs, and educational programs on nutrition.

Types of Research

Research on dietary components must concentrate on human nutritional needs in the developing countries and on the capacity of local foods and diets to meet these needs. The maximum safe intakes of given foods must be considered because of the presence of both naturally occurring and acquired toxic substances in many foods. Because of humid storage conditions, mold toxins are a particularly common problem. The effect of local methods of processing and preparing food on the nutritional quality of diets also must be determined. To formulate effective food and nutrition policies and educational measures, more must be known about local dietary beliefs and practices including traditional, religious, esthetic, and other values assigned to foods.

POLICIES AFFECTING NUTRITION

Until recently few governments have made any attempt to develop a coherent nutrition policy. However, many developing countries now have national planning bodies, and interest has increased in incorporating food and nutrition considerations into both sector policy and overall national planning. This has been strongly encouraged by such international agencies as the World Bank, FAO, the World Health Organization (WHO), and the new United Nations University, as well as by the U.S. Agency for International Development (AID) and several other bilateral agencies. The importance of nutrition planning has been persuasively argued but the necessary data base is extremely limited for most countries. Government policies that are formulated, implemented, and changed with little consideration for their ultimate effect on nutrition can nevertheless have major effects on nutrition.

Types of Research

One research area encompasses the nutritional effects of food supply policies and practices, including production strategies, agricultural research priorities, agricultural extension and rural credit services, food self-sufficiency, food aid, and resource use including land tenure practices. Another concerns the nutritional consequences of various food distribution and marketing policies and practices, including pricing policies, marketing technologies, delivery systems, international trade, and grain buffer stocks. A third research area would be the nutritional implications of general government policies, such as income redistribution, taxation, or employment.

Comparative studies of the experiences of different countries with particular types of policies are needed. Simple models need to be developed for predicting and evaluating the effect of program and policy interventions, which can be improved as knowledge is gained from their application.

Research in this area should examine the thesis that dietary requirements for sustaining good health, as measured by effects on human performance, are affected by changes in the social, psychological, and physical environment of the people concerned (see the report of Study Team 12). A corollary to this is that government action to reduce or offset the sources of stress in the environment can improve the nutritional status and well-being of populations.

Studies are needed of countries whose populations appear to be relatively healthy and nutritionally satisfied despite relatively low per capita levels of food consumption and income. Where such countries and regions exist (Sri Lanka and the state of Kerala in India are likely cases), are particular patterns of social and economic policy responsible for the results? To what extent can we attribute the quality of health and nutrition to such things as widespread health or educational services, egalitarian income and employment distribution policies, social policies that increase feelings of security, and mobilization of community energies in popular activities?

Such studies also can advance widespread efforts to measure the effects of development on the quality of life. Such indicators include more than gross national product and combine social, health, and economic variables to suit each case.

The role of women in determining family nutrition requires special attention. Most government policy fails to take into account the social and economic importance of women in the food system. Ordinarily, women select and prepare foodstuffs for the family. In the developing countries, women have a major influence on crop selection, particularly crops that will be consumed in the family or village. These influences and the role of women in shaping the physical and social environment of the home affect the nutritional status of the entire family. How well women perform these roles depends in part on their own health and psychological well-being.

NUTRITION INTERVENTION PROGRAMS

While it is true that the occurrence of malnutrition is largely determined by the socioeconomic circumstances of the individual or family, specific intervention measures can alleviate or even solve some nutrition problems without the time and resources required for social change. The classical example is the elimination of endemic goiter by the use of iodized salt in many countries. More recently, Guatemala has initiated on a national scale the fortification of sugar with vitamin A. Also, several Asian countries have begun to distribute massive oral doses of vitamin A to young children. Both interventions are designed to prevent blindness due to avitaminosis A. Iron deficiency anemia also should be amenable to direct intervention if suitable staples and methodologies for iron fortification can be identified.

Other types of direct intervention programs include nutritional rehabilitation centers, food distribution or supplementary feeding programs, and nutrition education. Programs of this type have been widely utilized by both the developing and high-income countries and have received extensive political and economic support. Unfortunately, an effort has seldom been made to evaluate their effectiveness.

The failure to evaluate adequately ongoing nutrition intervention programs makes it difficult to determine the effectiveness of past investments in nutrition and alternatives that might be considered in the future.

Many intervention programs have most certainly not been cost-effective and for economic and logistic reasons have not reached more than a small proportion of the vulnerable groups for which they were intended.

Types of Research

The research program would include developing and testing evaluation methodologies (determining what to measure, how to measure it, and how to interpret the findings for purposes of decision making). The research would test the evaluation methodologies in direct food distribution, fortification, nutrition education, and various health programs. Such research is essential for formulating nutrition policy and for designing nutrition programs.

POTENTIAL EFFECTS OF APPLIED NUTRITION RESEARCH

Substantial progress in improving nutrition should be possible by: (1) identifying questions to be addressed in choosing among intervention alternatives; (2) organizing current information around these questions and identifying gaps; (3) filling some of the gaps, at least tentatively, by short-term and medium-term research projects; and (4) experimenting with processes for formulating and executing plans and programs that will improve nutrition.

It is difficult at this stage to estimate the long-term effect of the recommended research. However, we know that improved diets can be a major factor in enhancing human well-being. Changes in diet may well turn out to be beneficial to the health and life expectancy of large population segments in the United States. In developing countries, effective nutrition interventions are likely to have more of an effect on human health than comparable investments in medical care.

Progress in the recommended research areas will depend on continuing and strengthening other types of research, including: fundamental research in the biological, behavioral, and social sciences, currently supported by the National Institutes of Health (NIH) and the National Science Foundation (NSF); direct studies on nutrition–disease relationships, family consumption patterns, and effects of dietary adjustments on animals, currently supported by NIH and USDA; research and development by the international research community on such projects as inexpensive nutrition surveillance techniques to identify groups and individuals most at risk; and early warning systems to alert planners to impending famine or acute malnutrition in vulnerable populations.

The proposed research will require many additional workers in the United States and developing countries with fresh perspectives and new skills, particularly to integrate the natural and social sciences into studies of nutritional status. Interested persons should have the opportunity to build these skills by combining research and operational experience. International cooperation can help compensate for the shortage of qualified researchers. The findings produced by such collaboration should be applicable to many countries.

The application of research results to achieve beneficial change will depend largely on decisions by governments as to what public policies they adopt and how much they spend on them. The current U.S. expenditure of about $80 million per year is largely used for nutrition studies with experimental animals or hospitalized patients. A new dimension of human nutrition research including social and policy factors is required. Study Team 9 estimates that a minimal nutrition research program would cost the United States approximately $20 million more annually for the first five years.

Food Production

Research on food production can find the technical means for improving average yield, stability of yield, product quality, and the efficiency of food plants. The low-income countries of the tropics particularly face difficult problems in achieving self-sustaining farming systems that produce high, stable yields with a minimum dependence on energy and capital.

Changes in plant performance result from research on plant breeding and farming practices. However, the potential for such advances depends on progress made on basic studies of biochemical, ecological, and biophysical processes and their genetic bases. The experimental yields of the leading crop research centers are approaching the limits of current knowledge gained from such basic research and are likely to be further constrained unless scientific and technological capabilities are harnessed more fully.

U.S. research has been concerned largely with temperate zone plants and ecologies, but the United States is capable of conducting more research relevant to the tropical ecologies of the developing countries. Some important differences exist, such as length of days, but the United States has a wide range of relevant ecologies within its own borders, including tropical and semitropical areas, high altitude or dry areas similar to parts of the tropics, and sizable areas of soils similar to soils in the tropics. The United States also has some of the same pathogen problems as the developing countries. More importantly, the United States is particularly well equipped to conduct research on generic traits and on genetic manipulation techniques that are transferable across plant types, and to undertake developmental breeding of improved plants in major crop species. Regional and local efforts in the developing countries could then fit these advances into crops and farming systems for other ecological zones and specific locations.

Each country needs to follow different commodity priorities. The United States can seldom tailor its research effort to the various situations found in the developing countries except by providing research assistance directly to these countries. We should not assign research resources to work in the United States on whole food plants that are not significant for U.S. agriculture when the work can be done better in the developing countries. However, more research should be conducted on the U.S. crops and varieties that are closest to those of the developing countries. This effort and a concentration on improving the general functional traits of food plants will increase the prospects that U.S. research advances will be incorporated into developing country practices.

There is another reason to increase U.S. attention to functional research priorities. U.S. yield increases have been slowing down. Many observers believe that this may be due in part to the excessive orientation of U.S. agricultural research to specific commodities and in part to the preoccupation of the basic biological research community with biomedical research. Whatever the causes, it is clear that work on the biophysical processes that control plant production has been seriously neglected.

PLANT BREEDING AND GENETIC MANIPULATION

During this century, scientific advances have enlarged our ability to develop new crop or animal strains tailored to the needs of particular regions or to special uses. Among the more obvious examples are high yielding hybrid corn and sorghum and the semidwarf varieties of wheat, rice, millet, and barley. Equally dramatic progress has occurred in the improvement of vegetables, some fruits, and the oilseeds, and in pasture and forage species.

It is now possible to adapt more crops to regions with short growing seasons, high or low temperatures, adverse soil characteristics, and inadequate rainfall. There have been changes in nutritional, storage, and harvesting properties. Most important, major increases have occurred in the productivity of many crops resulting from: the creation of highly efficient new strains; the improved and increased use of fertilizers and water; better disease, insect, and weed control; and the improved abilities of farmers to combine many components into highly productive farming systems.

The new crop and animal strains are the product of highly developed breeding capabilities. These have resulted from our increased understanding of the principles of genetics and of the genetic system of the individual species.

During the past three decades, when the United States has been more concerned with crop surpluses than with the need to increase production, less work has been done on plant breeding because of inadequate public financing.

During recent decades, scientific developments have occurred that promise to extend our ability to alter plant, animal, and other organisms to make them more useful to society. These developments include the transfer of basic genetic material from one type of organism to another, which could eliminate the constraints that genetic relationships impose upon the classical breeding methods. There also have been advances in cell culture and in mass replication of whole plants through tissue culture, among others.

Types of Research

U.S. research support should be increased in three areas: plant breeding and "classical" genetics, cell biology, and genetic stocks. This research will be furthered if scientists in this country and abroad who are working in these areas collaborate, together with those working in related fundamental scientific fields.

Plant Breeding and "Classical" Genetics   Particular attention should be given to the genetics of each major crop species, especially to the extent that a lack of basic genetic information on any species limits advances in plant breeding. Research should include work on forage and pasture species because of their importance for animal production and the potential contributions of such species to U.S. agriculture.

Special attention should be given to developing crop strains tolerant to stresses—drought, excess soil moisture, extremes of heat and cold, toxic factors in the environment, and deficiencies in soils (see "Resistance to Environmental Stresses," a separate research priority).

Mutation breeding, which failed to live up to previous expectations partly because of lack of knowledge at the cellular level, deserves serious reexamination as a genetic technique.

Classical genetic methods operate on whole plants, using selection of the better performers in the field. Thus they are essentially trial-and-error processes that rely on the chance production of desired combinations of characteristics that can be assessed only by time-consuming and expensive processes. If it were known which biochemical and biophysical processes in the plant determine the performance sought, the selection procedure could be shortened drastically.

Cell Biology   Recent research offers the prospect of a new level of genetic manipulation that could enlarge the capacity of conventional techniques to test and improve whole-plant yields.

Research along two principal lines is needed. First, there should be further development of ways to produce genetic changes at the cell level, and to stabilize these changes in whole plants. This research includes transferring genetic material between cells, and using cell fusion and/or introducing recombinant DNA. The U.S. government, in cooperation with the scientific community, is currently establishing controls to minimize the risks associated with certain aspects of recombinant DNA research. Substantial capital will be required to construct laboratories that meet containment standards.

The second line of research is to develop new methods to screen germ plasm for agronomically important traits. This may be accomplished at the cell level faster and more cheaply than with classical breeding techniques, if important cellular processes affecting yield or other performance characteristics can be recognized.

Although the primary goal is to improve the research techniques used for genetic manipulation of food plants, such work also will produce advances essential for other research areas discussed in this section, including biological nitrogen fixation. This work also will give scientists new research skills that will be useful elsewhere. A major effort is essential on this important research area.

Funding for current U.S. research activities of this type, which lags behind those in Europe, is estimated at less than $2 million annually. This level of expenditure does not approach realization of U.S. scientific capabilities. Considering the vast potential of this research, funding should be increased substantially.

Genetic Stocks   Scientists need access to stocks of genetic material (germ plasm) with the widest range of variability. Much of the existing diversity resides in wild or seldom cultivated plant or animal communities that are not in breeders' stocks. Techniques developed through the first two lines of research will permit improved analysis and conservation of genetic variants that would otherwise remain lost or unidentified. Offshoots of the same techniques will permit the efficient storage of disease-free germ plasm, thereby lessening the effect of plant quarantine provisions on the worldwide movement of genetic materials.

Collection, storage, classification, and retrieval systems for plant germ plasm should be developed on an international basis. The International Board of Plant Genetics Resources has recently launched such a program. While the United States has long been a leader in such work, the recently established National Plant Genetics Resources Board should encourage expansion of U.S. activities in the field of plant germ plasm, benefiting not only the developing countries but also the U.S. farmer and consumer. International exploration for potentially valuable new species and work on the conservation of natural habitats that have especially diverse floras should be part of this effort, in cooperation with the International Board.

Potential Effects of Research

We suspect we are nowhere near the limits nature has put on plant productivity. New techniques of genetic manipulation will permit us to achieve much greater productivity.

By accelerating classical breeding and genetics research, more varieties of plants would be available in the near future. New varieties based on genetic changes achieved at the cell level probably would not be available for another 20 years. However, research at the cell level can provide more immediate results to strengthen classical breeding, such as more rapid and efficient screening of plants for desired characteristics, and improved stocks of genetic materials. It is likely that such new techniques will permit combining of traits from plant species that could not be hybridized by conventional breeding methods and will offer other possibilities for altering whole-plant characteristics. These techniques will permit tailoring plants to specific performance needs more closely, quickly, and inexpensively than is currently possible.

BIOLOGICAL NITROGEN FIXATION

Nitrogen is a key element in the growth of plants and animals. Increased use of chemically fixed nitrogenous fertilizers has supported increases in yields over the past 25 years. Although about 45 million tons of such fertilizer nitrogen are used annually, this amount still is only about a third of the amount of nitrogen fixed biologically each year by micro-organisms. Biological fixation of nitrogen has not been increased substantially in recent years, but it is reasonable to believe that it can be increased. This should be a prime research goal.

If we have to rely entirely on increased use of chemically fixed nitrogen to achieve needed crop production during the next 25 years, the world production of fertilizer nitrogen would have to be expanded by two- to fourfold. One estimate suggests that 500 additional large-scale fertilizer plants would be needed over the next 25 years. At current prices, these plants would cost approximately $50 billion.

Shortages of natural gas and oil and the rising costs of these and other raw materials used to produce chemical fertilizers may constitute a greater constraint than capital costs on expanding fertilizer production. Research on biological alternatives to chemical nitrogen fixation is promising, and also offers a means of reducing the environmental con- tamination caused by nitrates and nitrites. The current annual U.S. ex- penditure on research on biological nitrogen fixation is about $4 million. The U.S. scientific community has the capabilities to expand its research effectively in this area.

Types of Research

Research to increase biological nitrogen fixation should concentrate on seed and forage legumes and cereals and other grasses as they are the predominant sources of calories and protein for the world's population. Seed legumes merit strong attention because most of the current bio- logical nitrogen fixation in agricultural lands occurs through symbiotic associations between leguminous plants and microorganisms. Increasing the amount of legume-associated fixation is a more immediate prospect than increasing the amount of fixation associated with cereal crops. Research with legumes may furnish information that can be later applied to the development of nitrogen fixation in cereals.

Increasing biological nitrogen fixation in legumes should increase crop yields and the monetary return per hectare. This should motivate farmers to plant more legumes in place of grains and root crops. This in turn will strengthen multiple cropping systems.

Some of the promising lines of research for increasing biological nitrogen fixation are: improving the current symbiotic association of leguminous plants and microorganisms; inducing microorganisms to perform a similar symbiotic role with cereal grains; and eventually, perhaps, transferring the genetic capability for nitrogen fixation directly from bacteria to plants. This last prospect eventually may have the largest payoff, but it depends on the new technology of recombinant DNA transfer. Although this work is encouraging, technical obstacles must be overcome, and transfers of DNA and dissemination of modified plants must be undertaken with caution. Research on biological nitrogen fixation, like research on other plant traits, should include an assessment of the interactions of modified plants with the ecosystems into which they are to be introduced.

In the Orient, nitrogen-fixing blue-green algae, living free or associated with water ferns, have been used to furnish fixed nitrogen to crop plants, particularly rice. It may be possible to utilize such algae to furnish nitrogen to a much wider range of crop plants.

In Chapter 3, we recommend a federally sponsored center to collect, evaluate, store, and distribute strains of bacteria useful in nitrogen fixation, and to monitor and seek to improve the quality of legume inoculants. The private sector should be encouraged, through means discussed in Chapter 3, to augment the research developed from expanded public support.

The success of research on biological nitrogen fixation may depend on progress in photosynthesis research. Photosynthesis provides the energy needed for nitrogen fixation, which in turn competes with other food-producing activities in the plant for the available energy. It is little appreciated that biological nitrogen fixation, like chemical fixation, is very energy demanding. If corn or other grasses are induced to fix nitrogen without corresponding increases in energy availability, it is possible that gains in yield would be less than gains from the equivalent use of nitrogen fertilizer. However, the process would have the great benefit of substituting solar energy for energy from fossil fuels.

Potential Effects of Research

Study Team 1 has estimated the potential effects of research on biological nitrogen fixation by cereal crops. If cereals could fix nitrogen at 25 kilograms per hectare or 30 percent of the rate at which the study team estimates soybeans fix nitrogen, the additional nitrogen fixed would equal 36 million tons. This amount is more than five times the consumption of fertilizer nitrogen in the developing countries. Extrapolating from current yield data in the developing countries, this amount of biologically fixed nitrogen could produce 200 million tons of grain, more than half the current output of the developing countries (excluding China). Benefits would be proportionally larger in the developing countries, which can afford less use of chemical fertilizers.

Even if we discount these estimates, the potential is huge and the need to accelerate research is urgent. Legume production probably could benefit from this research within 10 to 15 years, but it would probably require 15 to 25 years of effort to substantially apply the results of the more fundamental work, particularly on grains. Both USDA and NSF should expand their support of research on biological nitrogen fixation.

PHOTOSYNTHESIS

The lowest cost and perhaps the greatest potential for using the sun's energy lies in increasing the efficiency with which crops fix solar energy through photosynthesis. Most plants capture no more than 1 to 3 percent of the solar energy they receive. Present knowledge suggests a theoretical maximum capture and conversion of 12 percent. The main research task is to learn how to increase significantly net photosynthesis per hectare of farmland and how to direct the increased material that would be created into edible food products (or, perhaps, into fuels).

Types of Research

Classical plant breeding for higher yields has been responsible for changes in plant characteristics that increase net photosynthesis. For example, leaf structure and arrangement, growing periods, and life span can all be modified so that a plant can intercept more sunlight. Farming practices, such as increasing plant density so that more leaf area is exposed to sunlight or enclosing plants in greenhouses or plastic covers, also increase photosynthesis. These approaches need continued support. However, we emphasize more fundamental research that could bring sharp increases in net photosynthesis, particularly in economically valuable species. Better knowledge of the biochemical and physiological characteristics that underlie whole-plant traits, and new technologies of genetic manipulation, offer promising prospects for these investigations.

One such area of fundamental research involves inhibiting the processes that cause most crop plants to lose a large portion of the carbon dioxide with which they make plant materials. Certain plants, like corn and sugarcane, have natural mechanisms that suppress "photorespiration" (the light-aided consumption of stored foodstuffs) or that make these plants use stored material more efficiently in the dark. By studying these mechanisms, we may be able to improve photosynthetic performance and reduce the inhibitory effects of oxygen on net photosynthesis.

Another area of research might enable us to transfer useful traits from the limited number of photosynthetically efficient plants to the larger number of relatively inefficient food plants. Important properties include the rapid transport of photosynthetic products to storage regions of the plant, delay in plant aging, and the separation of cellular structures involved in respiration from those involved in photosynthesis.

These efforts have not been a major component of U.S. research on plant biology, although we have the scientific capabilities to pursue them. The interdependency between these efforts and the work on biological nitrogen fixation has already been cited. U.S. efforts should be increased within the next few years.

Potential Effects of Research

Study Team 1 estimates that there could be a 100 percent gain in yield in the tropics by slowing photorespiration and achieving greater oxygen resistance in the principal crops (excluding corn and sugarcane). They also estimate that gains of 25 percent or more in crops everywhere are possible by improving the efficiency of dark respiration. They anticipate that these and other routes to increasing photosynthetic efficiency could produce gains of 50 percent to well over 100 percent after 15 years of research at the level recommended.

RESISTANCE TO ENVIRONMENTAL STRESSES

The principal causes of instability of food output are a series of stresses on plants such as pests, weather aberrations, short-term droughts, temperature extremes, aluminum toxicity and related nutrient deficiencies of acid soils, and salinity. Research on pests and weather aberrations is considered as a separate priority research area below.

Most research has been designed to change plant environments in order to eliminate or moderate stresses. The strategy has been very successful, but would be costly if applied in vast areas of unused but potentially productive land.

Types of Research

The following seven areas of research to reduce the vulnerability of plants to stress should have high priority:

- Studying the morphological, physiological, and biochemical differences between susceptible and resistant varieties of the same species in order to make a sharp distinction possible early in the life of the plant. Success in this endeavor would lead to rapid screening techniques for identifying desired germ plasm and for selecting new varieties in a breeding program.
- Incorporating resistance to the conditions of acid soils, particularly aluminum toxicity, into new, higher yielding varieties of crop plants exposed to such stresses.
- Breeding crops for a shorter growing season to utilize the periods when drought or frost is least likely, and to allow for planting a substitute crop, if early crop failure occurs.
- Breeding for deeper and wider root penetration; extensive root development permits crops to use more of the scarce water and mineral nutrients in the soil, thus increasing drought resistance. Breeding for root penetration, shorter seasons, and tolerance to aluminum toxicity complement and reinforce each other in overcoming drought. The capacity of some grasses to penetrate deeply into inhospitable soils may establish root channels that can be used by other crops.
- Improving the symbiotic relationship between soil fungi and plants. Certain fungi (mycorrhizae) associate with plant roots and in effect extend the reach and functioning of the roots resulting in greater absorption of soil moisture and mineral nutrients.
- Breeding for higher tolerance to salinity, making use of wild species or varieties as a base. This will permit higher yields in extensive irrigated and semiarid dryland areas where yields are now depressed and permit more extensive use of irrigation waters of inferior quality.
- Modifying farming systems so that stress is prevented or reduced. For example, shading by intercropping reduces high temperature stress on the lower crop.

It is possible to make progress in research on stress resistance through conventional breeding approaches, but the greatest long-term progress is likely to come from reinforcing these approaches with the new genetic manipulation methods described in the first research priority area above. This will permit better screening of plant varieties for significant stress resistance traits and diagnosis of the underlying biochemical and biophysical relationships. Desirable traits may then be transferable between widely separated species. U.S. research should play a major role in advancing and coordinating work in this area.

Some of this research calls for special facilities to permit root observation without disturbing the environment of the soil.

Potential Effects of Research

The research recommended above will have three major effects: (1) crop yields should increase and stabilize in large areas that are under stress conditions; (2) more efficient use will be made of increasingly scarce energy-intensive inputs such as fertilizer, lime, and water; and (3) land that previously could not be cultivated will become suitable for agriculture. Most of the effects on food production could not be expected for at least 10 to 15 years.

About 40 percent of the world's potentially arable soils, more than a billion hectares, are acidic types that contain enough soluble aluminum (or related compounds) to restrict crop growth. This condition affects between two-thirds and three-fourths of the land that could be brought under cultivation, many of which are located in humid regions and in the developing countries. It is reasonable to expect average savings of 1 or 2 tons of lime per hectare or production increases of about 1 ton per hectare as a result of developing crop tolerance for aluminum. For instance, recently in some typical acid soils in Brazil, an aluminum-tolerant variety of sorghum required only 1 ton of lime per hectare, as compared with the usual 6 tons needed to increase the sorghum harvest by 5 tons. If the more modest expectation mentioned above were achieved on only 5 percent of the acidic soils, several billions of dollars could be saved. The cost-effectiveness of such research must be established.

The gains from research on resistances to drought and other factors will come from forestalled crop losses and from new possibilities for using technological developments that produce higher, more stable yields. New technologies may increase *average* output over the years, but output may be susceptible to heavy losses in years of drought or when other stresses are high. Because poor farmers in the developing countries have inadequate financial and food reserves, they cannot afford to invest in farming systems that may fail under stress conditions. They, therefore, often prefer traditional lower yielding farming systems that are more resistant to natural stresses so that output is more stable. Thus we can expect that research that builds greater stress resistances into the high yielding, modern production technologies will increase the use of these technologies in the developing countries and bring the greatest benefits to poor farmers.

It is difficult to estimate the size of these benefits, although it is thought that farmer concerns over stress resistances have been a powerful deterrent to the spread of high yielding technologies in the developing countries. Data from India for the two drought years spanning 1965 to 1967 are an example of the potential benefits of drought resistance. These data indicate that the drought cut national production 15 to 20 percent; production on many farms was virtually wiped out.

Large gains also can be anticipated for the United States. Drought still takes a heavy toll of U.S. crops. In the United States, there could be major savings if we could increase crop tolerance to acidic soil conditions. There are wide-ranging acidic soils in this country and farmers must use lime and phosphorus to counter acidity.

PEST MANAGEMENT

Pests attack crops, livestock, and food commodities. Some also serve as carriers of diseases for humans and animals. They are biologically diverse, including fungi, bacteria, viruses, nematodes, insects and other invertebrates, weeds, rodents, and birds. In other sections of this chapter, research is recommended to deal with the postharvest losses of food and damage to livestock caused by pests.

The magnitude of crop losses from pests is not known precisely but, worldwide, it is estimated to average about a third of potential food production. The world's most important crop, rice, suffers the most loss from pests—perhaps 40 to 50 percent. Pest losses vary widely over time and space, so that average loss figures obscure regional outbreaks that can devastate the food economy of an area. Some losses have been so consistently large that certain crops of great nutritional potential are not grown in particular areas. Preemptive losses of this kind are not included in estimates of pest losses but should be considered in the planning for research on pest problems.

Our current technology has not been able to stabilize levels of pest control because the effectiveness of some pest control practices diminishes over time. For example, the increasing resistance of pests to pesticides has seriously eroded the effectiveness of chemical control of insects, weeds, and certain plant pathogens. Replacement of one pest that is sensitive to a chemical control by another pest that is not is a common phenomenon. The evolution of new biotypes of disease organisms can make previously resistant plants and animals susceptible to disease. For these reasons, pest control research necessarily entails a ceaseless search for new practices just to "stay even." This includes the search, now primarily in the private sector, for more effective and safer pesticides.

A recent study on pest control by the National Academy of Sciences, *Pest Control: An Assessment of Present and Alternative Technologies* (1975), presents comprehensive recommendations dealing with the institutional and scientific needs in this area. Study Team 1 endorses these recommendations and emphasizes its own general strategy for progress in several specific areas.

Types of Research

The recommended strategy entails selecting and applying integrated pest management techniques that fit particular pest, crop, and animal species, and socioeconomic situations. This approach includes ecological research to: (1) characterize the important pests and obtain realistic estimates of the damage that they do and how they do it (this deserves particular attention on an international scale); (2) establish management guidelines for deciding on the timing and nature of control action and which pests are worth working on (this can involve developing mathematical modeling techniques to integrate the several control procedures and handle the large amounts of data needed to make decisions); and (3) field test management systems for integrated pest control.

Integrated control emphasizes combining several tactics to manage pests. Crop production is often unreliable when it is based on a single method of pest control. Yield increases and yield stability are more likely to be achieved when the burden of protection is shared by a variety of control tactics systematically combined on the basis of sound ecological principles. Population dynamics must be studied within typical ecosystems to determine how pest fluctuations are related to interactions within the natural community and how specific interventions might alter the community dynamics. Integrated control methods must be adaptable to local production practices, economically and environmentally sound, and socially acceptable. They are needed for various sizes and styles of agricultural operations with different mixes of labor and capital.

A number of high priority research areas constitute the tactical dimension of needed pest control efforts. The first area, fundamental to successful pest management systems both in the high-income and developing countries, is cultural control—the use of agronomic practices that favor natural antagonisms to pests. Such practices include: crop rotation; fertilization, tillage, and irrigation practices; sanitation; use of pathogen-free planting stock; and management of crop residues and animal wastes. Research is needed to study, identify, and describe methods of traditional agriculture that are effective in controlling pests.

The second area of tactical research is selecting and breeding plants resistant to pests. This area would include: (1) systematically exploring and identifying resistant germ plasm; (2) greater understanding of the biological properties of pest organisms and how these properties interact with different genetic varieties of food crops; and (3) developing plant cell and organ culture techniques for use in plant quarantines, in selecting pest-resistant varieties, and in developing interspecific hybrids more resistant to pests.

Third, biological control (introducing organisms that prey on particular pests such as insect viruses and bacteria) deserves particular attention because it could perpetuate itself without heavy recurring costs. Insects and some weeds have been the traditional targets of biological control; further attention ought to be given to the control of pathogens as well. The major kinds of research on biological control include: searching worldwide for controlling organisms, improving release and establishment procedures, and developing management systems that use biological control in crop production.

A special case of biological control is use of male-sterile and autolethal methods for insect control. These techniques are highly specific for particular target pests, which makes them useful in schemes of integrated pest management, and desirable because of their comparatively innocuous effect on the environment.

Potential Effects of Research

Enormous amounts of major crops are lost because of pests. World food supplies could be substantially increased if such losses can be prevented. For example, if 20 percent of the current losses in rice were saved, about 180 million people could be fed from the approximately 45 million tons of brown rice that would be available. An estimated savings of 20 percent is a conservative goal. Gains also would accrue from improved stability of yields, which would encourage farmers to adopt new practices that would increase output in addition to innovations in pest control.

A large part of the need in this area is research to adapt known technology. Thus increases in yields of both plants and animals can be expected early. Application of biological control techniques on a large scale is a longer term prospect.

WEATHER AND CLIMATE

Fluctuations in weather and climate cause the largest variations in food production. Thus efforts to alleviate agricultural problems arising from these fluctuations are crucial. Droughts, unseasonably high or low temperatures, and severe storms all cause significant losses in food. Famines, caused most frequently by droughts and floods, have occurred somewhere almost every year since World War II.

For the purposes of this report, "weather" refers to events, such as precipitation and temperature, occurring within a two-week period, while "climate" is associated with events occurring over longer time spans. Research on climatic changes has evolved from the recognition that climate is much more than average weather.

Past climatic trends and deviations from them are well documented. In the United States, from 1955 to 1973, the climate was less variable and thus more favorable to crop production than during earlier periods. But there is no basis for expecting such favorable conditions to continue. Serious consequences are predicted from the droughts that occurred in the Great Plains and the West in the winter of 1976–77. The tenuous margin between food adequacy and shortage is due, in part, to unfavorable weather and climatic fluctuations. The worldwide effects of weather in 1972 substantially reduced world food reserves and increased food prices.

Strong national and international programs for climate and weather are needed. Because of the high costs of weather research, agencies undertaking this research should make the maximum common use of experimental design, equipment, and data. For example, the National Oceanic and Atmospheric Administration (NOAA), the National Science Foundation, and the National Aeronautics and Space Administration (NASA) participate in the worldwide Global Atmospheric Research Program (GARP). As another example, NASA and USDA cooperate on many programs, especially on improved crop production forecasts. USDA has used the advanced technology of the worldwide programs to improve its information system through research such as the Large Area

Crop Inventory Experiment (LACIE). Research by NOAA and the Air Force Environmental Technical Application Center relates estimates on Soviet crops to USDA estimates.

We urge support for the Global Atmospheric Research Program sponsored by the International Council of Scientific Unions and the World Meteorological Organization. U.S. annual funding for research and equipment for GARP is in the neighborhood of $43 million. Established as part of the World Weather Watch and endorsed by the U.S. Congress, GARP has the twin objectives of understanding the transient behavior of large-scale atmospheric fluctuations in order to increase the accuracy of weather forecasting for periods ranging from one day to several weeks, and the factors that determine global air circulation in order to develop a scientific basis for predicting climatic change. The GARP program consists of two distinct but related parts: (1) design and testing of a series of theoretical models of the atmosphere to permit an increasingly precise description of physical processes that link the weather of a given day or the average weather of a given month to that of a subsequent day or month, and (2) studies of the atmosphere to provide the data required to design theoretical models and to test their validity. A massive year-long global observation program is planned for 1978–79, to be followed in the 1980s by an expanded international GARP program to study the processes that influence climate change, both natural processes and those that result from human activity.

Disturbing indications suggest that over the next century use of fossil fuels for the production of energy might result in a build-up of carbon dioxide in the atmosphere sufficient to increase global temperatures on the order of 3°C, and by more in the polar regions. The problem is so important to food production and other activities that it calls for concentrated efforts during the next decade. Research is essential to understand better the global carbon cycle and the distribution of carbon dioxide in the atmosphere, oceans, and biomass, and to develop an ocean atmospheric model capable of simulating global circulation and radiant energy transfer.

An objective for the 1980s should be ascertaining the degree of climate predictability and, within those limits, developing techniques for monthly and seasonal predictions. Equally important would be information based on historical variability of climate to help predict future climatic changes.

We applaud recent legislation directing the Secretary of Commerce to prepare a study on the state of knowledge of weather modification. This should provide a base for developing national policies that would take into account the legal, social, ecological, international, and scientific implications of weather modification. We also are pleased that the World Meteorological Organization is establishing a carefully designed field experiment to determine the feasibility of precipitation enhancement. The benefits from even a slight increase in rainfall are sufficiently attractive that the potential for research in this area must be determined.

Types of Research

We give highest priority to two related areas of research that have specific agricultural objectives. We also encourage work in four other areas of general weather and climate research, especially where they have implications for agriculture.

Our first priority recognizes that agriculture must obtain and make better use of improved weather and climate information. The worldwide GARP program should be adapted to developing country needs where feasible. Improved predictability will aid both U.S. and developing country food systems. Research on the better use of information will have immediate use in the United States and increasingly important uses in the developing countries.

The purposes of such research are to: (1) use better the statistical techniques for estimating weather and climate changes including geographic variability; (2) develop better models for handling farm risks that use probability distributions for the various cost and benefit factors; and (3) improve management skills for dealing with the effects of weather variability.

We endorse the emphasis on management in the recent National Academy of Sciences study, *Climate and Food* (1976). Farmers have made important adjustments to climate over the centuries, but this can be done more systematically. Management programs can reduce both risks and damages caused by weather events. Such programs involve decisions on crop and acreage mixes, pest control, seedbed preparation and planting, interseeding, timing and amount of fertilizer application, and harvesting. Animal production also can be adjusted: livestock rations can be altered to accommodate temperature changes, and animals can frequently be moved to shelter. Farmers currently alter day-to-day management practices according to expectations about weather. Improved biological response information and more reliable statements about anticipated weather would enhance their management capabilities.

Our second priority is the improvement of analytical techniques for predicting the effects of weather on crops, recognizing that, in large part, agriculture must adapt to weather and climate variability. There must be a better understanding of the responses of plants and animals to weather and climate variables. The previously recommended basic crop and livestock research for breeding to withstand greater stress of temperature and moisture would indirectly help farmers adapt to weather or climate. The research recommended here concentrates directly on helping farmers adapt to weather and climate.

Research using statistical approaches to link meteorological variables with biological responses has relied on bioresponse models. These models must be made more dynamic. Biological response functions should be established for several research areas including: canopy radiation interception, photosynthesis, translocation, respiration, morphology, phenology, root development, soil–plant atmosphere dynamics, water status, and nutrient uptake.

To pursue both of these research priorities, improved national and worldwide climatological data bases must be developed. Weather information needed for various agricultural areas should be identified. We therefore recommend:

- adaptive research to assist developing countries apply the predictive models of GARP;
- U.S. information programs to provide farmers with weather and climate information, including an expanded National Weather Service Program;
- assignment by the U.S. Cooperative Extension Service of an agricultural meteorology specialist in each state to assist in applying the research findings in this area.

This entire program must be well coordinated among all agencies and must keep the final users of the findings in mind. Training programs must be expanded to provide adequate numbers of highly qualified people to carry out these activities.

We encourage support for four other areas of general weather and climate research with implications for agriculture: (1) identifying limits of weather and climate predictability; (2) within these limits, developing predictions for three time spans—one month to a season, 1 to 10 years, 10 to 100 years, as well as predictions of climatic variability, at least for a 5- to 10-year period; (3) assessing people's inadvertent effects on climate; and (4) assessing the potential for weather modification nationally and internationally.

Potential Effects of Research

The high-income countries must take the lead in this research, but it will have important effects worldwide. Most production in the developing countries is highly sensitive to weather, and the vulnerability of farmers in the developing countries to climatic disasters has been a factor in some of the most catastrophic events in history.

An estimated three-fourths of the potentially arable land in the tropics have limited production capacity due to insufficient moisture. Meteorological services are increasingly used in high-income countries, but have been used less in the tropics due to the lack of data and research.

The probability of success with bioresponse models is high since a strong, well-established base in plant and animal physiology already exists. Imaginative interdisciplinary research directed toward closing present gaps in biological response data could result in substantial model improvements within three to five years. Complex multilevel models could adequately simulate plant and animal responses in about a decade. Simulation applicable to tropical areas will take longer, but special tropical considerations should be built into ongoing research now.

The effects that managerial and probability research could have are impossible to estimate. Fundamentally, it builds on the basic biological research that is given high priority throughout this report. However, application of that research will often depend upon the research recommended here. The potential effect is not limited to agriculture in the high-income countries. Identifying the "lead indicators" of some aspects of climate such as the timing and strength of the Indian monsoons would facilitate many management decisions. For example, the Indian Meteorological Service has had some success in monsoon forecasting. The mean surface pressure over tropical South America during April and the May snow accumulation over the Himalayas were found to be correlated with summer monsoon rainfall distribution over India.

The effect of greater accuracy in forecasting would be substantial. Personnel and institutional support for this research should come through augmentation of the existing research effort. The resources required would be $10 million annually for at least 10 years. The agricultural benefits, though difficult to estimate, would be substantial.

The GARP program is not expected to benefit the developing countries for at least 10 years. In the long run, this program should significantly affect weather prediction in the tropics. The meteorological programs of many countries should be improved as they are coordinated into GARP. Countries involved in programs such as the Monsoon Experiment (MONEX) (e.g., India, USSR, and Japan) are already planning research to adapt the GARP results to their own regions.

The capability to anticipate climate anomalies would markedly help to manage food storage and distribution. The effect of climate is further illustrated by research on the relationship of climatic stress to protein content in rice by the International Rice Research Institute (IRRI).

We do not yet know enough to estimate what effects the four general weather and climate research areas we recommend would have on food production worldwide. However, we do know that research on climate and weather is vitally important, and, if successful, could have dramatic effects on food production in the future.

MANAGEMENT OF TROPICAL SOILS

Most of the potentially arable land that is not farmed is in the tropics of Africa and South America, about 1 billion hectares or three-fourths again as much land as is presently cultivated in the world. Seventy percent of this unused arable land has acidic soil belonging to the groups called oxisols and ultisols. Similar soils cover large areas of the United States.

In some tropical areas the climate permits production all year. There are encouraging indications that these two soil types, if handled properly, can produce high crop yields. However, growing conditions in many tropical areas are far from ideal, and much research will be required before cultivated crops can be grown economically and without affecting the environment adversely.

Types of Research

An approximate sequence of research needs is: (1) classifying local soil types and strengthening of research work in representative locations; (2) establishing suitable land-clearing techniques where applicable; (3) identifying low-cost, efficient methods of correcting deficiencies in soil composition which would be used in combination with new plant varieties that tolerate local stresses; (4) identifying economical measures to maintain good soil characteristics for water retention, root penetration, and other plant needs; (5) developing of suitable cropping systems and/or forage-animal systems; and (6) adapting emerging technologies and adjusting them to local ecologic and socioeconomic needs within specific development projects. Much of this research includes experimenting with cultivation practices for improving farming systems. Tropical soil research should include exploring natural soil–plant ecosystems to determine how they can best support new high yielding crop varieties with minimum reliance on chemical and physical amendments to the soil.

The soil classification work should be complemented by the development of a worldwide data base on soils that permits widespread, fast, low-cost transfer of information. The information should relate physical characteristics of soils, environmental conditions, and appropriate soil uses. The oxisols and ultisols discussed above and the wetland rice production regions should be high priority areas for classification.

U.S. work on soil taxonomy, including experiments with computerized storage and retrieval systems, provides a good base for developing a data system for worldwide use. Soil scientists outside the United States have contributed valuable help, and the data are already being used in many countries. U.S. research organizations also can help with the methodological components in the research described above, and they can exchange scientists with the developing countries to facilitate both site-specific and generic work. Although the needed research and development is site-specific, findings from similar areas can be widely transferable.

Potential Effects of Research

The potential of farming the unused acid soil areas of the developing countries is suggested by recent research in Africa and Latin America. Two or three crop sequences per year on ultisols with the moderate use of chemicals have produced yields per crop in those areas that are approximately 80 percent of yields in the United States. Annual crop production in those humid lands, if well managed, could be raised to 150 to 200 percent of temperate zone production per hectare. The much larger savannah areas of oxisols usually support only one crop per year without irrigation, but can produce year-round with irrigation. They also have the potential for increasing beef production.

Many of these lands now have a low population density and their development will involve extensive migration of people, both through organized schemes and spontaneously. Major commitments have already been made by some governments (e.g., Brazil, Peru) to open up substantial areas of land, and other countries may follow with similar policies. Unless such development is technically and economically sound, many enterprises will fail. This will result in a permanent loss of resources on the site, severe damages downstream, and social hardship as disappointed settlers return to their crowded places of origin. Managing acid soils with less use of lime and fertilizers is also increasingly important in the United States.

The difficulties of the research problems and of the settlement process suggest that the major effects of this research on production cannot be expected in less than 10 to 15 years.

IRRIGATION AND WATER MANAGEMENT

Adequate water is indispensable for plant growth. Having enough water depends not only on average annual precipitation, but also on the reliability of supply. Farming systems can be highly productive on relatively small annual supplies, if the supplies are dependable or if the soil adequately stores water in relation to variations in rainfall. Unfortunately, precipitation is the most variable and least predictable element of weather. Large regions of the earth experience variations of as much as 40 percent from their average precipitation. Despite ample average rainfall, three-quarters of the area farmed in the tropics is limited in productivity during part if not all of the year because of insufficient moisture. The water problem for world agriculture is, thus, not total water availability, but when and where water is available.

Today, 14 percent of the world's farmed area is irrigated and the percentage of food produced on irrigated land has increased substantially. Various estimates suggest that the area irrigated could be more than doubled. However, as most of the world's farmers will not have access to irrigation, there is also a great need for improved water management in rainfed agriculture.

Water use in irrigated agriculture is too often grossly inefficient. Known principles and techniques are not applied, often because of policy and institutional restrictions. Present practices frequently lead to waterlogging and salinization, which decreases productivity. More often they waste both water and energy and degrade water quality.

Research is needed to increase efficient uses of water, including research to adapt known principles and techniques to actual situations. Comprehensive programs in water management adapted to specific local conditions should be developed. Policy and institutional research needed in this area is mentioned in "National Food Policies and Organizations."

Types of Research

Two approaches to the water problem are generally applied, and we propose research priorities in both. One involves altering physical conditions to provide optimal water supply for maximum crop production. The other is concerned with adjustment of overall farm management operations to improve crops under varying conditions of water availability.

Research on physical conditions includes adjusting tillage and cropping practices so that soil can retain more moisture; improving irrigation technology and related work to improve drainage and salinity management; and improving watershed management to maximize water supply reaching the root zone of crops and to reduce erosion and soil deterioration on watersheds and cultivated land.

Research on irrigation should concentrate on providing crops with low-cost, efficient, uniform supplies of water. Attention should be given primarily to the farm field and the root zone of crops. In the developing countries, research should concentrate on small farm and community irrigation systems, including provision of supplemental or partial irrigation from groundwater or locally stored supplies, and on the need for managing such systems locally. There should be more opportunities for combining sophisticated concepts with simple technologies for practical application in the developing countries, e.g., computer modeling of the structuring and operation of systems to deliver water to farms, coupled with simple delivery systems at the local level; or use of advanced methods such as laser technology to survey areas suitable to land leveling, even where oxen could be used to move the soil.

Improvements at the farm level depend, in the case of larger water supply systems, on the ability of the farmer to obtain water at the time and in the quantity required. Thus an important interaction exists between centralized water management/planning and onfarm water utilization. The structure of an irrigation system can place severe restraints on the irrigator's options to apply sound conventional or innovative water management and practices. Plans are currently being prepared to extend irrigation to millions of additional hectares, and these plans should take into account the interaction between farm use and the water supply system.

Improvement of farm management operations should combine field experiments with plant modeling and systems analysis. An encouraging start has been made on techniques for computerized simulation modeling that will help to identify the most promising combinations of crop varieties, planting dates, plant population density, and water management practices to guarantee optimum use of available moisture. For the development of optimum management schemes, such research needs to be closely coordinated with work in breeding and genetics to select cultivars best suited to the environment. Although these techniques are still primitive, some early applications have already contributed to large improvements in yield.

The ecology of parts of the United States has much in common with that of the developing countries. The United States, therefore, has had much experience with water management research that is relevant to the developing countries. Further, it has accumulated substantial worldwide experience with these research problems, primarily in connection with AID programs. Thus it can do valuable functional work here that would be useful overseas, and can participate in international research networks to extend and adapt this generic research overseas through local research on farming systems or on irrigation and water management.

Potential Effects of Research

Three-fourths of the farmland in the developing countries is limited in productivity because crops do not receive enough moisture. Additional soil is lost through erosion and waterlogging. Improvements in water management could double yields over substantial areas. Small expenditures on research and development could produce large benefits, particularly for small-scale supplemental irrigation.

With this research, large investments in water resource development would be more likely to yield projected benefits, and could prevent losses of soil and water quality that are largely irreversible.

This area of research requires applied work that could produce results in the near future on a wide range of water problems that restrain crop production in the developing countries. Research could help overcome the management constraints placed on the farm irrigator by the social framework in which he or she operates, or by the lack of effective local organization. Larger improvements can be made over the longer run as the more fundamental research produces results. These would be valuable for the developing countries.

FERTILIZER SOURCES

The use of chemical fertilizers is usually the most rapid means of increasing farm production. In the tropics, nutrient deficiencies are particularly great (see also "Resistance to Environmental Stresses").

Results from research on biological nitrogen fixation may require as much as 15 years, and will not cover all crops and situations. Thus requirements for inorganic nitrogen fertilizers are likely to expand.

Two areas of research are recommended for developing new sources of fertilizers: (1) identifying less expensive methods of producing nitrogen fertilizer that do not use the increasingly scarce natural gas and petroleum that are the principal raw materials for current production, and (2) designing fertilizers that are most efficient for use in the tropics.

Fortunately, the United States has, at the Tennessee Valley Authority (TVA), the strongest fertilizer research capacity in the world. TVA also has had extensive experience in the developing countries. This experience provided the initial base for establishment of the autonomous International Fertilizer Development Center (IFDC), which is dedicated to work on the fertilizer needs of the developing countries. IFDC is located alongside TVA's fertilizer research facilities, permitting close technical cooperation between the two organizations. These two institutions could lead the research recommended below.

Types of Research

Several high priority lines of research are recommended for providing more economical sources of nitrogen fertilizer.

Research is needed on new methods of producing ammonia, the base of fertilizer nitrogen. The most promising approach for replacing the current production process is to develop an improved process for producing ammonia from coal. Study Team 4 thinks that U.S. research in this area has a high probability of success and would provide a 25 percent reduction in energy use for ammonia production.

Another technically promising route is to improve processes for converting waste hydrocarbons to ammonia. However, there are doubts about the cost efficiency of this procedure, particularly for large-scale production. This may become a useful approach for small-scale production in developing countries lacking coal, petroleum, or natural gas. U.S. interests are likely to expand because of growing waste disposal problems. IFDC, AID, the Environmental Protection Agency (EPA), the Energy Research and Development Administration (ERDA), and FAO or other organizations providing assistance to the developing countries could collaborate in this area.

New means of producing hydrogen, a primary input in the production of fertilizer nitrogen, could eliminate dependence on conventional hydrocarbon sources. Processes involving hydrolysis of water may have some appeal in locations where enough low-cost energy and water are available to permit economical use. Other processes, although possible, have shown only limited promise.

In the long run, it may be possible to develop an industrial process to draw nitrogen from the air and produce ammonia under natural pressures and temperatures. This would emulate biological nitrogen fixation and would be a major scientific and technological breakthrough. Because of the tremendous effect this line of research could have, the exploratory phases of fundamental research to determine its feasibility should receive stronger U.S. support.

The second major area of research is the formulation of new types of fertilizer needed for the tropics. Aside from nitrogen, the most important current need is lower-cost sources of phosphorus. This mineral is particularly needed for productive farming on the acid soils predominant in the developing countries. Rock phosphate can sometimes be substituted for the highly processed phosphate fertilizers generally used. Current industry standards for phosphorus, based on experience in the temperate regions, may need to be modified for the use of phosphorus in the tropics. The current methods of production are effective on 15 to 20 percent of the world's known phosphate ore reserves and frequently use only 40 percent or less of the phosphorus in this ore. Better processing methods must be developed to permit use of a larger percentage of the known reserves and to increase the recovery percentage. IFDC, in cooperation with scientists in Brazil and other places, is giving this work top priority.

Large areas of the tropics often lack sulphur and a variety of micronutrients, which need to be incorporated into mixed fertilizers. Requirements for individual nutrients in the developing countries differ from country to country. Fertilizers should be designed to release nutrients slowly, thereby providing plants with nutrients throughout more of the growing cycle and preventing the loss of nutrients caused by leaching. Fertilizer could then be applied less frequently and in smaller total amounts. One important goal is to reduce the amount of nitrogen lost to plants from evaporation or from leaching. One-half to three-fourths of the nitrogen in fertilizers is dissipated in this way. It has been estimated that evaporation depletes the nitrogen in world soils by 120 million tons annually, almost three times the amount of nitrogen applied in the form of chemical fertilizers.

Research on the better provision of plant nutrients must combine proper use of fertilizer sources with alternative strategies, several of which have already been mentioned. Another important strategy is the recycling of organic wastes. Only by effectively combining all strategies can we provide a long-term, stable source of plant nutrients with a reasonable dependence on exhaustible mineral and energy resources.

Potential Effects of Research

Research to improve methods of producing nitrogen will be particularly valuable for the coal-rich countries that currently, or that will, import large amounts of petroleum or natural gas, e.g., the United States and developing countries such as India, Pakistan, and Bangladesh. Success is probable within 10 years, given the current technology base.

The advantage of converting wastes to ammonia is the substantial and rapidly growing supply of this raw material for the production of fertilizer nitrogen.

Developing an improved industrial process, which uses less energy, to draw nitrogen from the air may be the ultimate solution. If exploratory results confirm the feasibility of this process, research in this area should become a major U.S. priority, involving both government and industry, with possible collaboration by other countries. Large commercial applications are a long-term prospect.

Success in developing better fertilizers for the tropics would lower the costs and increase the effectiveness of fertilizers used in the developing countries and also has U.S. applications. Such research will probably produce a series of modest successes that, cumulatively, will influence food production substantially in the developing countries.

RUMINANT LIVESTOCK

Animal products are a major part of the world's diet. In the United States, livestock produce two-thirds of the protein, one-half of the fat, one-third of the energy, four-fifths of the calcium, and two-thirds of the phosphorus for human consumption. In the developing countries, animal products are a much smaller though still important part of the diet—they provide 10 percent of the calories and 20 percent of the protein.

Animals increase the supply of food for humans by consuming resources that otherwise would contribute little to feeding people. These include forages from grasslands and other ranges, plant by-products, cellulosic wastes, crop residues, and browse. These resources are best suited as feeds for ruminants such as dairy and beef cattle, water buffalo, sheep, goats, llamas, alpacas, and wildlife. Other resources are best suited for swine and poultry. These include roots, nuts, insects, vegetables, fruit crops, garbage, animal wastes, animal by-products, plant by-products, and plants with only moderate fiber content. Edible coarse grains may be used by all livestock and poultry when the supply of these grains exceeds that needed by humans. In some countries, small animals such as guinea pigs, rabbits, and game animals eat certain feed resources not used by humans. Crop production will continue to yield inedible plant materials acceptable for animals. On most croplands almost half of the total digestible energy of the plants is left after harvest. Two-thirds of the world's agricultural land is in the form of permanent pasture, range, and meadow, of which about 60 percent is not suitable for cultivation. Food processing and industrial wastes also can be used by animals.

Animal production has increased rapidly and can be increased even more. Animal production can play a more important role in the developing countries, but great care is needed in devising range management systems that avoid overgrazing or other ecological problems.

Most of the world's potentially arable land that is not farmed is in the tropics. However, it will be a long time before most of this land can be cultivated productively. Other huge land areas, suitable only for grazing, are best used by ruminants, especially by beef and dairy cattle which now produce almost half of the world's meat products and most of its milk products. Cattle are the dominant ruminants in the United States. Therefore, research on these ruminants should benefit both the United States and the developing countries.

This research also can result in some U.S. input into worldwide research on other ruminants, such as sheep, goats, and water buffalo. These and small farm animals such as swine, poultry, rabbits, and guinea pigs need to be considered in research on farm systems in the developing countries.

Types of Research

Research should simultaneously pursue improvements in three areas: (1) forage production for ruminant livestock, and other related means to upgrade wasted or underutilized materials; (2) animal health; and (3) animal genetics and reproduction.

The improvement of forage and ruminant livestock requires a well-planned, interdisciplinary approach. Improvements in animal health and genetics can result in better utilization of feed. Conversely, better feeds improve disease resistance, health, and reproductive rates. Beyond their value as feed, improved forages are an important means of increasing soil fertility. ·

In the developing countries, research is needed on the selection and improvement of forage plants, especially tropical legumes that can spread rapidly on tropical ranges and pastures and provide more digestible energy and protein. Greater use of trees and shrubs should be considered. Forages provide all but a small part of the feed for livestock in the developing countries and over half of the feed for ruminants in the United States. Forage research should be coupled with experimentation on ecosystem management, on both small and large ranges. The natural and socioeconomic factors found in the principal grazing areas also should be considered. Forages may provide the ground cover needed to reduce soil erosion. Rangeland carrying capacity can be greatly increased by improved legumes and grasses and the use of better management practices.

As noted in the sections, "Resistance to Environmental Stresses" and "Management of Tropical Soils," many tropical soils are acidic. Thus basic and applied research on the genetic tolerance of forage plants to these soils will be of value for animal production, as will some aspects of research on pest control. For example, insects reduce livestock efficiency and cause disease, and weeds reduce feed efficiency.

Research on contagious animal diseases is critically important for livestock programs in the developing countries. Epidemic disease control should be supported by research on the socioeconomic effects of the various diseases and on disease control procedures, including infection of humans. Some animal owners may resist using measures to eliminate animal diseases, and there are other difficulties in implementing control procedures in the developing countries. But this area has demonstrated benefits. Some of the endemic disease research being undertaken in the United States will have worldwide effects, especially in the longer run.

Genetic research on livestock should concentrate on developing superior animals that can consume low quality diets and that are more resistant to disease. This work should expand ongoing research on genetics, nutrition, and reproduction physiology, and should seek the higher net product return gained by increasing the number of offspring per head of breeding stock. Research also should be undertaken on improved feeding and management at critical times in the life cycle.

All types of research, from fundamental to applied experimentation, are required for animal production. Not as much fundamental research on animal problems has been conducted in recent years, but it should receive increased funding.

Multidisciplinary teamwork and coordination between plant and animal research are necessary for solving most of these problems. International research collaboration should integrate knowledge provided by U.S. research facilities, the international agricultural research centers, and the national programs in the developing countries. Personnel in the developing countries must be trained. USDA should seek to coordinate U.S. support for this research, support which should be increased, including support of the AID-sponsored consortium of U.S. universities.

Potential Effects of Research

Research on ruminant livestock and forage will permit us to capture one of the world's largest wastes of potential food supply. This expansion need not compete with land needed for grain production. Increasing the availability and digestibility of lignin and cellulose for ruminant livestock could increase ruminant output in some developing countries by 25 to 50 percent. Complementary to this would be improvement in the nutritive value of indigenous feedstuffs. For many nations this could result in a 20 percent improvement in animal performance. The United States has a substantial stake in this research. Improved forages can help release grain for human use and expand acreage available for food production.

Research on animal diseases could ultimately result in opening up large new areas of production. Approximately 700 million hectares in Africa, capable of supporting 125 million cattle under good management, now support only about 8 million cattle because of the prevalence of trypanosomiasis. FAO estimates that the developing countries lost 30 million tons of milk and 15 million tons of meat and eggs from animal diseases in 1970—and this is a conservative estimate. The United Kingdom spent $425 million eliminating an outbreak of foot-and-mouth disease in 1968. A similar outbreak in the United States, if it remained uncontrolled, would cost $10 billion in a year, according to USDA estimates. The elimination of some animal diseases also could eliminate some of the same diseases that affect humans.

A recent case illustrates the potential of research on animal diseases. A successful U.S. vaccine against Marek's disease in poultry was used worldwide following its development in 1969. In the United States, it reduced condemnation losses in broilers from 1.57 percent in 1970 to less than 0.25 percent in 1974. Over the same period the mortality rate of layers was reduced by 14.8 percent. The return on the research investment for this vaccine has been estimated at 220 percent per year.

Improving animal health in the developing countries could reduce the danger of importing animal diseases to the United States. Diseases have prevented imports of animals and animal products and have inhibited the international exchange of animal germ plasm and the introduction of new breeds of superior livestock.

Research on genetic improvement in livestock would make it possible to implement new programs and to upgrade existing ones substantially. The development of highly productive milk animals in the lowland tropics should result in annual increases of 500 to 1,000 kilograms of milk production per cow within 10 years. The United States has doubled the level of milk output per cow within the last 25 years. Crossbreeding

Zebu with Criollo (native) cattle in Latin America has already increased pregnancy rates and carcass weights by at least 15 percent, and this figure can be increased substantially. Estimates are that nearly 50 percent of the potential numbers of animals of the major livestock species in the United States and other high-income countries are lost because of low reproductive performance, prenatal and postnatal mortality, and poor management. Losses in the developing nations exceed those in the United States.

Animal production often can be developed faster than new land can be developed for crops. This helps open up new settlement areas which gradually include more cropping. Forage production may also improve the fertility of these areas. Cattle also can provide agricultural power and fertilizer in mixed farming systems and can convert agricultural residues to food.

Animals are an important stockpile of food and capital for the developing countries. The total caloric worth of worldwide animal stocks in 1974 was 50 percent more than that of grain stocks, and the former were more evenly distributed.

In addition to providing nutrients directly and supporting of rural and industrial development, this research could increase personal incomes and foreign exchange earnings for several low-income countries.

AQUATIC FOOD SOURCES

Fish are an important component of total human and animal food intake. They are equivalent nutritionally to meat in protein, low in saturated fats, and high in essential minerals. Fish are culturally acceptable in areas suffering from malnutrition where there are cultural inhibitions to the use of other animal foods. At least 750 million people in the Pacific basin, Southeast Asia, the Indian subcontinent, and coastal Africa and South America derive 50 to 85 percent of their animal protein from fish harvested from coastal zones, estuaries, and fishponds.

In 1974, the world commercial production of food products from fresh and saltwater was about 70 million tons, excluding whales and seals. About 86 percent of this came from oceans, and the remainder from freshwater. About 5 percent of the total consisted of shellfish. Five million tons were obtained from aquaculture or fish farming, mostly in freshwater.

Until 1969, the annual rate of growth of the world catch from marine fisheries was nearly 8 percent. Between 1969 and 1975, the annual growth rate fell to slightly more than 2 percent, largely because of a decline in the Peruvian anchovy catch. Although some of the contributing factors may be temporary, there is also overfishing of some stocks and increasingly damaging pollution in certain coastal areas. The catch of many major commercial ocean species is at or near its sustainable maximum.

However, the world catch could be increased by the development of capture techniques and markets for some underutilized stocks such as herring-like species, squid, and unused stocks like krill and deeper swimming fish. This would require costly technology. It is estimated such technology could result eventually in a fourfold increase in catch. However, there is the possibility that oceanic food chains would be affected adversely. The high-income countries in the temperate regions would benefit primarily from this effort rather than the food-short nations of the developing world.

In several regions of tropical seas, the upgrading of traditional fishing and processing methods could lead to an additional harvest of 20 to 30 million tons which could be used directly in countries now suffering from hunger and malnutrition. This would require little production research but realization of the gain would depend on technical and social research on the processing and distribution of the new harvest and traditional catches.

Optimally, developing aquatic food sources faces unique and difficult management problems. The seas are a common property resource that increasingly will come under national management. However, many stocks of fish cross national boundaries; thus effective management requires regional as well as national institutions. The United States has a great deal of expertise in the management of international fisheries, derived from its pioneering work with commissions and treaties. Therefore, the United States should be able to assist the developing nations in interdisciplinary work on policy problems concerning the development of aquatic resources and management.

Types of Research

Fisheries and aquaculture differ. A fishery is essentially a gathering of wild animals, whereas aquaculture employs varying degrees of direct animal management. Applying research to increase aquatic animal production is promising in both of these areas.

The first major priority is to reduce waste and to upgrade the final product through processing. Twenty-nine million tons of the 1974 commercial catch of 70 million tons of aquatic products were converted to fishmeal and oil. At least 20 million tons of the world catch are wasted in processing fish for human consumption. That leaves about 20 million tons or less for direct human food. In addition, close to 10 million tons of secondary or by-catch fish are discarded by the fishing boats. It is estimated that shrimp fisheries alone will produce 10 to 20 million tons of such by-catch by 1985.

To make fuller use of the world fish catch, we must: (1) improve methods of pick-up and transfer of fish at sea, (2) preprocess by-catch species on shipboard, (3) process fish currently used for conventional fishmeal to extract proteins for high-grade animal or human food, (4) upgrade portions of fish now underutilized in order to formulate prepared food items for direct human consumption, and (5) develop intermediate processing technologies that are particularly applicable in the developing countries. Technologies to reduce spoilage of the highly perishable fish products are needed at all stages. This work is aimed primarily at marine fisheries, but parts of it would reinforce the development of aquaculture in fresh and brackish waters.

The second major priority involves two lines of research on aquaculture:

– A long-term research effort to improve the breed and supplies of seed stock of aquatic animals should be undertaken, concentrating on tropical or semitropical locations. However, basic science support could be provided elsewhere. The principles of genetic selection have been applied to a few species found in the temperate zone and recently to tropical species through the controlled spawning of grey mullet and rabbitfish. Research in other countries has resulted in the controlled spawning of marine shrimp. Reproduction in these species can now be sufficiently controlled to permit studies of selective breeding. In the near term, however, the foremost task is improving the survival rates of offspring. The ultimate aim is to produce breeds of marine animals that are superior in growth, resistant to disease, adaptable to local conditions, and that show hybrid vigor. Beyond straightforward selective breeding, other more sophisticated genetic manipulations also appear to be technically feasible.
– Research also should be undertaken to improve the uses of managed waters in the tropics, mainly for polyculture (the growing of several compatible species of fish in a single body of water or enclosure). It is expected that polyculture will eventually become the primary mode for the cultivation of aquatic animals in the fresh and brackish waters of the tropics.

Much of the research for the expansion of fish production through aquaculture must take place in the production areas themselves, and to this end a number of national and regional research centers have been, or are being, established, in many cases with help from international sources. The United States has a great deal of competence in basic and applied animal nutrition, including fish (for example, Auburn University has had wide experience in the developing countries with research, technical assistance, and training in aquaculture. Some of the U.S. experience in animal genetics and breeding could be applied to research on fish. With support from AID and perhaps from the Departments of the Interior and Commerce, these U.S. capabilities could contribute significantly to international collaboration on research and development.

Facilities for research on aquatic food sources should be established at one or more of the existing centers that have access to local deliveries of fresh fish, extension and training facilities, and the capabilities for fishery or aquaculture research.

U.S. centers with such capabilities should be linked with the appropriate centers in the developing countries. A number of institutions could participate in this research: the National Marine Fisheries Service and the Sea Grant Program in the National Oceanic and Atmospheric Administration, the Department of Interior, AID, FAO, the International Development Research Centre of Canada, and the International Center for Living Aquatic Resources Management (ICLARM), a Rockefeller-initiated, nonprofit research organization located in the Philippines.

U.S. research and technology capabilities also could be applied, albeit at an exploratory level of effort, in several areas of aquatic food production, such as: (1) aquaculture associated with the production of electric power from the temperature differential of surface and deeper layers of water in tropical seas, a prospect now under scrutiny in the United States (deeper waters are rich in nitrates and phosphates, which are conducive to aquatic animal husbandry); (2) the selection for ranching, through the appropriate hatchery operations, of species that could be sent to pasture in large artificial lakes as well as in the ocean inside and outside the 200-mile extended economic zones; (3) the application of satellite technology for locating schools of fish; and (4) the development of bioengineering devices for herding and/or capture of fishes by means of light, sound, or scent. Research in these areas can take advantage of technology development that will proceed for other reasons.

Potential Effects of Research

Research that would enable a fish catch to be used more fully could produce results within a fairly short period of time. These results would be useful both to the United States and to the developing countries. The newly established 200-mile offshore jurisdictions, which extend the area in which countries have exclusive fishing rights, make investments to increase production in these areas more worthwhile.

Research could greatly reduce the extent of the global waste of fish catch. It is estimated that the amount of fish protein directly consumed by humans could be doubled without increasing the present world catch. Technically these developments could take place within the next decade.

Research on aquaculture will raise yields over time. Study Team 3 estimates that the annual yield of pond fish in Southeast Asia could be raised five times its present average of 600 kilograms per hectare through polyculture coupled with improved nutrition. This potential combined with the growing interest of the developing countries in aquaculture, both at the village level and in large commercial operations, promises substantial gains.

Genetic improvement will permit larger-scale gains needed in the longer run. The breeding potential of tropical aquatic species has scarcely been tapped; therefore, some early gains can be expected. Fish geneticists estimate that selective breeding alone could soon increase production 2 to 5 percent per year. Advances made in breeding milkfish, mullet, and tillapia, for instance, could eventually result in the production of several million additional tons of these and similar fish. Such increased production would greatly benefit the poor who live in Indo-Pacific coastal areas. Indeed, the world has not begun to realize the potential inherent in the genetic improvement of aquatic animals.

FARM PRODUCTION SYSTEMS

A major problem constraining the use of new technology by farmers in developing countries is that technology usually comes to them, if at all, in disconnected pieces. Thus they have difficulty fitting it effectively into their farming and social systems. Research on how those systems are constructed is of high priority. Since farming systems involve many factors, the research must be multidisciplinary. The perceptions of those people in the system who affect farming practices, such as farmers, village leaders, and managers of governmental and private services, are important factors to consider.

Often traditional farmers have, through centuries of experience, developed great skill in agriculture and animal husbandry within the bounds of the technologies available to them. The approach to increasing their production must begin with understanding what traditional farmers do, why they do it, and the results that they produce. Much can be learned from their experience and skills. Modern research should be used to explore ways to improve their production and income.

It is important to recognize the wealth of resources often found in the tropics. In Nigeria, for example, one may find single communities that cultivate more than 50 plant species that comprise their food supplies. As new farming systems are introduced, the value of these riches in terms of dietary variety, seasonal distribution, resource utilization, and ecological equilibrium must be maintained and enhanced.

Two common constraints are important in shaping farming systems. First, small farmers in developing countries often cannot finance large amounts of purchased inputs and their ability to do so will increase only gradually as their farms grow more productive and market conditions become more favorable.

Second, labor problems are complex. In some rural areas, even though there is large-scale underemployment, labor shortages may occur, particularly in planting and harvest periods. Traditional technology has contributed to poor living standards and to large-scale suffering in many rural areas. The backbreaking work, accompanied by nutritional inadequacies and an unsanitary environment, has made rural life undesirable to many, and they seek escape in the cities.

Improved farming systems in most developing countries should be relatively labor-intensive due to the shortage of capital and under-employment of labor, particularly where labor/land ratios are high. Innovations are needed to reduce the onerous aspects of farm work, to spread work more evenly throughout the year, and to use the year-round production potentials of the tropics to their maximum advantage. Such improved systems, however, should not become heavily dependent on purchased inputs.

Research on farm production systems has excellent prospects for greatly increasing production, income, and social well-being. It should include:

- selecting crop combinations with regard to effects on total income and nutrition;
- introducing improved varieties of crops and animals that permit higher yields, increased annual production per farm, and more stable incomes through adjustments in the length, timing, and mixture of growing seasons;
- preserving the diversity of species and protecting soil resources for long-term production;
- experimenting with crop combinations, sequences, and improved cultivation techniques that will keep the need for purchased inputs low;
- designing equipment to meet the needs of small farmers for tillage

and other cultivation, irrigation, farm storage, and crop handling;
– improving the organization and administration of local services;
– improving the management skills of farmers and housewives needed for the production, preservation, and consumption of food.

Natural and social scientists should collaborate to tailor these possibilities to the realities of the farmer's socioeconomic environment.

Research on farming systems at the International Institute of Tropical Agriculture (IITA) in Nigeria and at the International Rice Research Institute in the Philippines suggests that such work can bring large production and associated nutritional, income, and ecological benefits. For example, IITA is experimenting with systems that use a permanent green ground cover and no tillage. Two crops (one cereal and one legume) are planted through the ground cover three times per year. Complementing these biological technologies are specially designed types of light equipment that are inexpensive, use little energy, and are easy to manufacture, operate, and maintain. Results include tripling of annual yields, improved soil fertility and moisture retention, reduction in soil erosion, improved weed and other pest suppression, lower inputs, elimination of the heaviest labor, and spreading of labor requirements much more evenly over the year.

Other farming systems are being designed at the International Crops Research Institute for the Semi-Arid Tropics (ICRISAT) at Hyderabad, India, to meet the environmental stresses encountered in the semiarid tropics where there may be alternately too much or too little water. The emphasis is on "water harvesting," monitoring the water balance, and evolving systems that maximize the productive use of labor, fertilizers, improved crop varieties, and the many other improved technologies available.

U.S. domestic circumstances are beginning to stimulate new interest in research on a number of the same problems that are common in the developing countries, especially with small farms. Examples include: reduced tillage coupled with herbicides for weed control to conserve energy and soil and to reduce the need for pesticides; reduced use of other high-cost and high-energy inputs; new types of multiple cropping, and the engineering of crop varieties to fit new multiple cropping systems; and the recycling of organic matter.

Types of Research

One line of research is the improvement of methodologies used to identify farming systems that are well adapted to the local ecosystem and socioeconomic environment (see the report of Study Team 4). Comparative analyses of existing traditional, modern, and mixed systems are needed to establish what works, what does not, and why. Systems research is providing new analytical tools that can be applied to complex problems in this field.

Research also is needed on multiple cropping systems including improvements in the plant and animal components, in cultivation practices, and in pest control and other stress resistances. The purpose is to achieve farming systems that satisfy such goals as expansion of output and income, food security, and nutritional improvement. Farming systems also should provide for conservation.

Research is needed on: interactions among crops growing together and sequentially; interactions among plants, soil, water, and animals (sometimes including fish); recycling of organic matter through the system; effects of all this on tillage and other cultivation practices; interaction of the whole on pest control; and other critical factors. Studies should not be restricted to the traditional crop species, but should include a wide variety of plants, including trees, in carefully balanced and well-integrated production systems, including those on small farms. Diversification of crops and animals contributes to food security for the family, locality, and nation.

Research on farming systems may identify desirable characteristics of crops and livestock that have been neglected in prior research. Characteristics can be identified that have production, nutritional, and marketing advantages for local systems and for work on improved varieties.

Soil and water management is another important research area for particular farming systems. Systems built around zero or minimum tillage are especially important in the humid areas of the tropics. The objective is to maintain or enhance soil tilth and fertility and to use the available water resources more effectively, reducing the fluctuations in crop production from season to season.

Work also is needed to develop equipment to make multiple cropping systems feasible and to improve labor use. A need exists for inexpensive, easy-to-operate equipment appropriate for use in the tropics. Such equipment can be designed, as the work of IITA and IRRI illustrates.

Changes in the farming systems of developing countries can improve the status of women and children. Frequently women and children contribute much of the labor on the farm but receive relatively small shares of the gains. Farming systems and institutional arrangements that reduce drudgery, give women better access to services such as credit for their own farming enterprises, or release children for more education would bring great social gain.

The types of research needed are location-specific, but the United States can contribute in several ways. This country is experienced in methodological research and farm management economics. The developing countries are short of skilled people for farm-level empirical analysis. The United States can provide methodological training and specialists who are needed for farming systems work in the developing countries.

U.S. agricultural and social scientists also could be assigned to work in the developing countries as a part of local teams. USDA scientists could participate in this undertaking in the context of the international mandate proposed in Chapter 3.

The United States should support international research collaboration on farm management systems. A small but promising start has been made by several international centers and by some U.S. institutions. This work should be expanded.

Potential Effects of Research

Food production on currently farmed land in the humid tropics can be increased, perhaps by as much as fourfold in the long run. The introduction of new farming systems, requiring minimal resource inputs, should play a vital role in this regard. Substantial but more modest increases in yield per hectare seem likely from improving farming systems in the semiarid tropics.

Farming systems in the developing countries also would benefit from a continuous flow of results from the fundamental and applied research suggested earlier in this chapter.

Food Marketing

The importance of research on food production and nutrition is widely accepted. Less accepted or appreciated has been research on the problems associated with food marketing. Yet, research on the marketing, processing, preservation, and distribution of food could result in reduced food costs and could stimulate both production and consumption, particularly in the developing countries. The kinds of research necessary vary widely among countries and are related to such factors as state of technology, extent of urbanization, level and distribution of income, size of country, nature of the production and consumption systems, and distribution of population. The research must be flexible and often oriented toward adaptive work.

The quantity and quality of food available to consumers depend in large part on the efficiency of a chain of services linking production with consumption. The chain can be short, involving only the farmer and household members; intermediate, as in the farm-market system in which farmers bring their produce to local marketplaces; and long, as in the complex marketing systems of the high-income countries.

Most farmers in the developing countries produce some part of their output for sale, and do not produce all the food they consume. Thus the efficiency of food marketing plays a major role in even the least developed countries and rural areas.

To improve the quantity and quality of foods consumed in the developing countries and the real incomes of producers and consumers, a number of improvements are needed in the marketing chain:

- reduction of waste;
- reduction of costs;
- better maintenance of food quality, or enhancement by fortification or other processing;
- wider and more even distribution of supplies over time and space;
- better communication of consumer demands to producers.

The lines of communication between producers and consumers are particularly poor in the developing countries. Farmers would produce more and different kinds of food if they were better informed about consumer demand, and consumers would buy more and different kinds of food if they were available.

Another characteristic of marketing in some developing countries is the predominant role of women in the processing and trading of food. Research must take this characteristic into consideration. Often the role of women extends beyond selling in the local market to operating large-scale, sophisticated marketing services, e.g., the wide-ranging marketing trucks of West Africa. In many areas, female entrepreneurs may need only modest encouragement and opportunity to expand and improve distribution and processing.

The U.S. food marketing and distribution system is complicated and advanced. Marketing services absorb about two-thirds of the average consumer dollar spent on food. This system requires continuous research on advanced technology, basic food science, and the policy, regulatory, and economic problems of marketing. Some information from U.S. research, when properly adapted, can be used by the developing countries.

U.S. marketing technology is largely in the hands of private enterprise whose entry the developing countries are often reluctant to accept. Thus there are special problems in making U.S. research skills in marketing available to the developing countries. The policies and inclinations of the developing countries in this area must be considered, together with the regulatory policies that most governments have affecting the incentives of farmers, the structure of markets, and the role of private enterprise in improving marketing technology.

U.S. research could benefit from participating in work on some of the food marketing problems in the developing countries. We recommend two research areas: reducing postharvest losses and expanding markets.

POSTHARVEST LOSSES

Decomposition can set in as soon as food is harvested. It is estimated that in some parts of the world as much as 50 percent of the food supply from plants and animals is lost between harvest and consumption. In humid tropical climates, the problem is acute since food deteriorates rapidly and refrigeration is inefficient, costly, and scarce. We need to know more about the magnitude and nature of these losses. Technology must be relatively low-cost, simple, and easily applicable in rural areas if it is to be effective among the poorest populations of the world.

Types of Research

The most important immediate research task is to establish more accurately what the losses are by commodities, by country, and at different levels in the marketing chain. Research then must determine whether these losses are attributable to poor management, inappropriate pricing and policy, or lack of needed technology. Lines of research and development that promise the most improvement at the least cost then could be chosen, both for the high-income and the developing countries.

AID and other development assistance agencies have already undertaken some of this exploratory work on postharvest losses. Three lines of research seem especially promising.

First, efforts on preharvest pest control should be extended to the postharvest phase. Similar technology can be applied, but new elements such as inexpensive and pest-resistant containers become more important as the food moves closer to markets. The development of new packaging materials is important.

Second, technologies for food preservation in the humid and arid tropics should be improved, particularly for use at the farm and village levels but also for urban use. One approach is to modify traditional or new technologies now being used to make them work better. Because women are most often responsible for the preservation of food, research workers should learn from them the methods they use. Women should also collaborate in the development of any improvements that can be made.

Local methods can be supplemented by new technologies created by food and materials science. Technologies that should prove useful include partial dehydration, fermentation, use of solar or other energy sources for preservation, and even in some cases more energy-costly microwave methods combined with airtight packaging and storage. Plant species that are genetically resistant to particular types of deterioration also should be investigated.

Extending the life of perishable products by three or four days, without the use of refrigeration, would improve the family diet and greatly expand the market radius for farmers in the developing countries. Furthermore, food products must be preserved for longer transportation routes and longer time periods.

Third, food storage must be improved. Bacteria usually cause spoilage, but huge losses are also attributable to pests and rodents, spillage, pilferage, and water damage. Research in this area also should consider partial processing.

This research can be carried out both in the developing countries and in U.S. laboratories (including the Defense Department's Natick Laboratory). AID could contract for ongoing U.S. research that could be adapted to the needs of the developing countries and could help to create research relationships between U.S. researchers and food science laboratories in those countries. NSF, USDA, and others should support fundamental research on the biochemical and physiological processes involved in the deterioration of animal and vegetable products.

International collaboration on research in food preservation is becoming important. Research in the high-income nations is being pooled by a recently formed group of international donors who will explore postharvest technologies, including those for reducing losses, in the developing countries. The new United Nations University is planning research, in cooperation with other universities and institutions, on better conservation and use of food already produced.

Potential Effects of Research

The size of the savings in postharvest losses can be appraised more accurately after an initial inventory of the losses is made. An inventory may seem a modest start, but it will identify the needs and direct efforts more efficiently. A study currently being undertaken by the National Academy of Sciences, "Postharvest Food Conservation," will provide some of the needed information.

Problems of food preservation in the developing countries have diverted production away from the more perishable products and toward those that keep well under tropical conditions. Such practices poorly serve the needs for better nutrition, higher incomes, and more productive mixed farming systems. Thus effects would go beyond the obvious food savings. Spinoffs useful in the United States also can be expected.

MARKET EXPANSION

When farmers in the developing countries increase their production, the market must be sufficiently large to absorb the increased output. Moreover, farmers often must be assured of markets before they will adopt more expensive production inputs that will increase their yield. The expansion of markets can stimulate production as well as handle increased production once it occurs.

There are two approaches to expanding markets: (1) increasing the purchasing power of the consumer, especially of the poor consumer who needs food; and (2) increasing the number of outlets for products by developing new uses or forms of products, new market areas, and new institutional arrangements.

Expanding markets can provide consumers with a wider variety of foods at lower cost, and can reduce the losses of food that result when supplies that accumulate cannot reach markets. Research is needed to reduce the physical impediments to the movement of food supplies and/or the lack of information that cause market imbalances.

Types of Research

One major area of research for the developing countries is how to enhance the purchasing power of the consumer, especially that of the poor consumer. Some practices used to make food more available to the poor include: (1) food-for-work programs, with at least part of the wages paid in food; (2) price-controlled stores or depots for foods in low-income neighborhoods; and (3) government-subsidized foods. Thus far there has been little research to assess the efficiency of such programs, and more research is needed. Research on U.S. food distribution systems may be useful to programs that try to solve some of the same problems in the developing countries.

Studies of demand elasticity also are important. Most such studies in the developing countries have been carried out in urban areas and limited in commodities covered. Studies of household consumption should be carried out in both urban and rural areas. They should encompass all socioeconomic groups and cover major commodities. Most studies have been concerned with markets that are little used by the poor. Thus how the very poor respond to changes in prices and incomes is another area that needs to be studied. Research also should be undertaken in the developing countries on how to shift consumption patterns to more nutritious foods.

Research to develop new products must be encouraged for the long run in the developing countries. Traditionally, those countries have marketed products that have had little processing. Extraction processing has become popular in some developing countries. This technology has been applied to rice, oilseeds, and sugar, and new markets for products have been found.

Food processing can provide needed employment and improve the product line for export to the high-income countries. Research is needed on the relationship of processing improvements to other factors affecting market expansion, such as improved handling systems, market facilities, and methods of transporting farm products.

Markets that serve small holders are frequently no larger than the distance the farm family can walk to and from a local village. Extending the radius of the local market often is the best means of increasing the incomes of farmers and others in the food system. Linking local markets with regional, national, and international markets further extends the marketing radius.

A number of factors limit the size of the market. The limitations of transportation are probably the single most important constraint, followed by food preservation and storage.

U.S. research could help the developing countries improve transportation systems, including better location of services for different stages of marketing. Research also is needed for the design and engineering of better modes of transportation, including vehicles that can extend the local farm-to-market radius. For example, research could develop sturdy, low-cost, all-purpose automotive vehicles for local manufacture; balloon or ropeway transport for local and regional movement over difficult terrain; and improved use of air freight for international markets.

Research could provide better options for strengthening local and regional marketing institutions, not only as centers for food exchange but also as service centers that provide for transportation, storage, and preservation of food. Systems should be designed to synchronize food production and its inputs with handling, processing, and transportation facilities. Organizations involved in food marketing in the developing countries should be studied. These include government, private firms, and cooperatives that can provide small farmers with market information and technical services and local processors with information on intermediate or possibly final processing. Case studies and comparative evaluations of marketing organizations could be used to identify experiences that can be transferred throughout the world.

Research on intermediate marketing institutions should include consideration of the role of women in food distribution and consumption. Women require technical and scientific training to enable them to work with local women in the developing countries in order to tap and upgrade their skills.

Success in improving intermediate marketing organizations greatly depends on the commitment of local resources and time. Marketing must be closely coordinated with research on production. Most marketing research must be done in the developing countries, but U.S. researchers can help design and evaluate research methodology.

Another research priority is applying modern analytical techniques to the planning, organization, and management of commodity flows in the developing countries. This work should identify bottlenecks in producer-to-consumer flows, and improve communication in the system. Systems analysis of commodity flows could be applied to these problems. AID has initiated research in this field among U.S. organizations and management research and training institutions in some developing countries. Such joint research efforts should be expanded.

Potential Effects of Research

Large amounts of food are lost in the developing countries after the food leaves the farm. Improvements in marketing could prevent much of these losses, and could help the developing countries even out the distribution of food over areas, seasons, and years.

This research would stimulate food production and provide better nutrition for more people. In so doing, it would lay the foundation for evolving larger and more productive food systems in the developing countries. The results of this research should be evident within 5 to 10 years.

Policies and Organizations

Science and technology alone cannot improve the world food and nutrition situation. Government policies and the organizations affecting food must provide incentives and opportunities for increased production and better distribution of food for people in the developing countries. Unless there are adequate price policies, farmers will not increase production; without adequate incomes, the poor cannot purchase enough food to meet their nutritional requirements. Hence research on social and economic policy is essential.

Some low-income countries, such as Taiwan and Sri Lanka, have developed a variety of policies and organizations that operate relatively effectively in their societies. These policies have contributed to increased food production, lower death rates, and reduced birth rates.

We are learning that in countries that suffer from a scarcity of land and overpopulation, small farms are not less productive per unit of land than large farms. At times they may even be more productive. Because small farms are more labor-intensive, they provide more people with the income necessary to buy food. Large mechanized farms, in regions such as northern Mexico, have contributed to a growing number of underemployed, landless workers.

Illustrations of the effects of national policies and organizations are plentiful. Technology that permits farmers to grow more food at a lower cost per unit of output can be offset by government price, tax, or trade policies that influence the prices of farm products and inputs. These policies can make increased production unprofitable for producers, thereby discouraging use of the new technology. For example, artificially low food prices intended to help poor consumers may result in lower production, and thus contribute to food shortages. Policies that favor expanding output but disregard consumer income are shortsighted. Policies affecting agricultural production may encourage the replacement of nutritious food crops with less nutritious crops or with nonfood crops, so that farm income and dietary adequacy move in opposite directions.

Inadequate credit and marketing services affect the dependability of supplies of seeds, fertilizer, and machinery, and may discourage farmers from applying improved technologies. Credit and marketing organizations in the developing countries often discriminate against the smaller farmers who till most of the land. Policies that limit access to land, water, or fishing grounds further reduce productivity.

International policies and organizations are of great importance to the world food supply. World grain production dropped 3 to 4 percent during the bad weather years of the early 1970s. Primarily because of inadequate trade and stabilization policies and organizations, prices increased by several hundred percent and the poor could not buy enough food.

Poor countries would have more incentive to apply better technology in food production if they had more opportunities to expand sales into international markets, particularly sales of products for which they have a comparative advantage. But policies and organizations often restrain such efforts. Trade policies for food have become increasingly liberal in recent decades, but many farmers are still deprived of potential sales worth billions of dollars and many consumers are faced with higher food prices because of poor policies and organizations.

The list of policy and organizational problems is long, and the specific content and relative importance of each differs according to time and place. This section identifies some of the highest priority research areas that are needed, but first we must stress two points.

First, experience suggests that the developing countries often have common problems regarding their policies and organizations affecting food. Comparative analysis of the experiences of different countries could result in widely applicable generalizations that would help each country adjust its own policies and organizations to its own unique situation. The United States can contribute to this effort. It can work with researchers in the developing countries to build simultaneously the knowledge base and research capabilities.

Second, the amount and difficulty of the research needed on policies and organizations will require a large increase in current social science research capabilities, both in the United States and in the developing countries. Social science research on food and nutrition lags significantly behind that of biological research because of shortages of skilled personnel, suitable methods of research, data, prior research findings, research funds, and effective organization. The situation is the most serious in the developing countries. Until these shortcomings are corrected, we cannot expect significant results from research.

NATIONAL FOOD POLICIES AND ORGANIZATIONS

National policies and organizations and their efficiency vary widely. They grow out of different cultures, political processes, resource endowments, and many other factors. Research is needed on the nature of these differences and on ways to improve policies and organizations.

Types of Research

One important line of research would determine the important cause-and-effect relationships among variables underlying human performance in food systems. This includes: how risk and uncertainty affect decision making behavior; which factors cause farmers and agribusiness firms to save, invest, and disinvest; which factors determine the choices consumers make among foods; and which behavioral factors underlie interactions between social environment, health, diet, and human performance.

Important methodological questions for fundamental research include how to measure nonmonetary objectives and values, how to develop interdisciplinary research teams, and how to monitor the effects of various policies and programs on the underlying behavioral variables found in the rural areas of the developing countries.

The second line of research would examine how policies that affect income distribution also influence food production and nutrition. Some areas that should be examined include: changes in land ownership or tenure; alternative approaches to increasing rural and urban employment; alternative policies affecting access to and the content of education; rules on water rights, fishing rights, or grazing privileges; changes in the rights and roles of women and children; and changes in access to the political process or to public services such as credit and health.

A third important line of research involves comparative analysis of national organizations with common functions. It would be valuable to learn why some organizations succeed and others fail and to identify ways to improve their performance. Such studies should examine three groups of institutions: those that provide analytical support for government policymakers; those that build and transmit knowledge on food and nutrition (research, education and training, extension and communication); and those that provide services and inputs to farmers and rural populations (e.g., credit, marketing, physical inputs). These service organizations are sometimes called "intermediate organizations" because they link the rural communities with the larger world around them.

The highest priority for increased U.S. support to organizational research is for studies on:

- the effects of different degrees and types of centralization and decentralization, or of local authority versus central control;
- the effects of different degrees and types of participation by local people in the various organizations that affect them;

- relationships between staff performance, types of training (including management training), location of training, and selective recruitment;
- the effects of collaboration among research institutions in the developing countries and international, U.S., and other high-income country institutions with common interests.

Methodological research on food sector analysis is the fourth priority area. This research would seek to improve techniques for gathering and analyzing the large amount of information needed to predict how alternative government policies and programs (or other events) might affect the various goals a developing country might have. This would require further development of systems work. For example, a country may be seeking to improve nutrition, to expand food output and exports, to increase employment and income, to stabilize internal affairs, and to improve its international status—all at the same time. What actually happens depends on how hundreds of factors work together. Governments that lack an understanding of the interdependencies within and between the agricultural and other sectors are usually forced to make uninformed choices among alternatives. The net effect of their actions often differs from anticipated effects and frequently actions work at cross purposes. With improved techniques for analysis, countries can allocate scarce resources more efficiently. Moreover, they can temper public expectations with realistic statements about what is possible.

Systems research, which has developed useful methodologies and equipment to handle large amounts of information, should be extended to strengthen analysis of food policies in the developing countries. Illustrative policy problems to which systems research could be applied include: choices among crops; the effects of alternative pricing and trade policies; management of commodity systems (production–marketing–consumption) at the national and international levels; decisions on the alternative uses of land and water; the effects of changing energy costs on production and consumption patterns; and the effects of alternative technology innovations, which in turn bear on research allocations.

These four research areas are ideal for collaboration between U.S. social scientists and those of many developing countries. The United States can contribute its methodological capabilities and intercountry experience to augment the skills of researchers in the developing countries. AID should expand its support for such work under Title XII.

The more fundamental research described in the first priority area would be appropriate for NSF support.

Potential Effects of Research

The potential effect of the research recommended above is open ended. The research often is important in giving direction to research in other disciplines, and, such research may help to synthesize the research of others. It directs policy and guides the formation and improvement of organizations. Errors in policy direction and organizational design are costly. Since researchers should be able to produce results early in the research process, such research can prevent many of these costly errors. This research can identify the areas in which data collection and analysis are essential and thus aid in the design of information systems. The greatest effects would come in releasing the energies and capabilities of many people now held back by poor incentives and limited opportunities. The cumulative effect over time will be large if U.S. research efforts concentrate on helping the developing countries build their own capabilities for work on policy and organizational improvements.

TRADE POLICY

The developing countries depend upon international trade in food and in the principal inputs used to produce food, such as fuel, fertilizers, and pesticides, to provide adequate food supplies for their people. The trade policies of both the developing and the high-income countries affect the ability of the developing countries to meet their goals for food supply, development, and nutrition. Conversely, policies on domestic food production and consumption directly affect trade.

There are many unknowns about the nature and extent of the interactions among the principal factors affecting trade. These unknowns limit the ability of individual countries to make rational choices on trade policies and impede productive dialogue on the international issues of increasing concern to all.

Research is needed to better understand patterns of world food production and trade that take advantage of the resources indigenous to certain areas and that will reflect the real costs of food production in various parts of the world. This research will improve the prospects for meeting the world's nutritional requirements more economically (including those of the United States). Research also is needed to anticipate technology and development trends and how they may affect the specialization of production and trade.

Although the developing countries must produce most of their own food supply, both those countries and the United States could benefit from expanded trade. For example, we both may gain from a trade pattern in which the United States imports a greater proportion of products more efficiently produced in the tropics (including such agricultural items as tropical horticultural products, sugar, and animal products), while developing countries import more products (such as grains) that are more efficiently produced in the United States. Such trade patterns can lead to increased real incomes and lower food costs for the countries involved.

Changes in trade or production patterns will necessitate socioeconomic and political adjustments. Research is needed to better understand the benefits and costs that arise as changes and adjustments occur.

Types of Research

We give high priority to three lines of research, which are elaborated in the report of Study Team 10.

The first line of research would identify the effects that would result if the high-income countries liberalized their trade policies for agricultural products from developing countries. A great deal is known about the different tariff and nontariff barriers to trade, but relatively little empirical information exists about the actual effects of these barriers: for example, the effects of trade liberalization on levels of production, distribution, consumption, prices, investment, employment, income, trade, and foreign exchange movements. These effects will vary by region, country, economic sector, and commodity. Research also is needed on the comparative advantage of areas or nations for producing commodities that are important in international food trade, and on how these advantages might be affected by technical assistance or international research collaboration.

The second line of research would analyze the consequences of different types of international management or regulation of prices and quantities of commodities involved in international trade. A growing number of such schemes is on the agenda for international negotiations over the next few years. Yet little research has been done on such major questions as:

– how international commodity agreements affect food availability, the use of resources, employment, prices, incomes, and trade patterns in producing countries;
– how the stability of commodity prices affects the stability of incomes and export receipts;

- how methods of commodity price indexing affect general price levels, real incomes, income distribution, and food availability, and whether improved methods of indexing can be developed.

The third line of research would develop analytical systems to help the developing countries determine the costs of meeting their commodity needs from the various domestic and foreign sources of supply, and what pattern of supply would minimize costs. One need is to develop and adapt simple models for quantitative analysis that can be used throughout the developing countries. Such models would be a useful framework for organizing and maintaining information on food production, consumption, and trade.

USDA should take the lead in advancing research in this area, drawing on its extensive experience in building trade models and in analyzing international commodity trade. USDA also should facilitate the participation of university researchers in this work.

Potential Effects of Research

The ability of the developing countries to cope with their food problems depends primarily on their success in sustaining a rapid rate of increase in food production. For most of these countries, world market conditions in food and related commodities will continue to be an important factor in their ability to increase their food production. We have seen that liberal trade policies can expand incomes, lower food costs, and increase access to production inputs. The present trade barriers are costly to the United States and the developing countries (see Chapter 1). Some recent FAO analyses suggest that free world trade in agricultural commodities would raise aggregate incomes in the developing countries by as much as $38 billion or 6 percent in five years, and export receipts by $10 billion. The staff at the World Bank estimates that if the United States, Canada, Japan, and the high-income countries of Western Europe removed trade barriers for nine agricultural commodities, export receipts of the developing countries would increase by $7 billion, and presumably would increase even more over time.

FOOD RESERVES

Food reserves can be an important means of minimizing the effects of unstable food production on human nutrition. Reserves consist largely of grains because they can be stored relatively inexpensively. Grains also can be transported more easily than other foods; thus they can be moved more readily to areas in which food production has been affected adversely by climate or other natural disasters.

Since World War II, the world has depended on grain reserves held primarily by the United States and other grain exporting countries for food security. Most countries have had access to these food reserves in times of need. These reserves have been backed by a relatively flexible production base that can respond to international market demands for additional grain supplies.

During the 1950s and 1960s, the large grain reserves held by the United States and other major exporters were not accumulated deliberately, but inadvertently as the result of farm income and price support policies. At times the reserves became so large that maintenance costs became politically unpopular. Efforts were made to reduce these grain reserves, including programs to limit production of the major grains. In 1972 and 1973, the major exporting countries tended to sell their stocks as rapidly as possible, and at relatively low prices. International grain prices increased markedly when it was realized that the major exporters no longer had excess stocks. Such situations as this are complex and policymakers need more information to help them manage stocks.

The experience of recent years indicates that without a clear understanding of how to manage reserves, the mere existence of large stockpiles of grain will not stabilize grain supplies and prices. The primary objective of reserves should be to offset part of the year-to-year variability in grain production and thus contribute to the stabilization of food supplies. Such an objective, if achieved, would have price stabilizing effects, although prices vary for reasons other than deviations in supply.

Grain reserves are expensive. Annual storage costs are about one-seventh of grain value at their recent levels. Thus, while food reserves can be valuable, the optimum size of reserves must be determined carefully. Because of the high costs of holding reserves, other means of minimizing variability of food supplies should be evaluated. These include international trade, the modification of government policies affecting domestic price stability that increase international price fluctuations, and the reduction of fluctuations in output. For the world as a whole, grain production varies relatively little from year to year. A large part of the instability of grain supplies in the international market is due to domestic and trade policies that limit access to otherwise available supplies.

Types of Research

Two principal lines of research have priority: (1) improving food reserve practices in the developing countries, and (2) exploring alternative means of stabilizing food supplies and their relationship to the operation of food reserves.

The first line of research would investigate the storage systems of particular developing countries. Relatively little is known about the size of their grain stocks, where stocks are held, who owns stocks, the losses during storage in the various types of storage facilities, and the costs and gains from storage, both within the year and from year to year. Research should first more accurately describe and evaluate current systems and then evaluate how these systems could be improved.

For both high-income and developing countries research should determine the effects of government ownership of reserves upon the reserves held by private individuals and firms. It may be that a large fraction of reserves held by the government simply replaces stocks that would otherwise have been held by farmers, consumers, and marketing agencies and that the size of government stocks may give a false sense of security. Price policies and international trade can reduce private incentives to hold stocks. The magnitude of these effects should be examined.

The second line of research would examine the alternatives to holding grain reserves. For an individual country, international trade may be an alternative: excess crops can be exported or imports can be reduced; or, if supplies of crops are small, exports can be reduced or imports can be increased. Research is required to determine under what circumstances international trade would be a more economical means of stabilizing domestic supplies than would holding reserves.

Research on national and international food reserves should consider geographical, technological, and policy factors that limit the access of food-short areas to sources of supply, or that limit the access of areas with surplus foods to possible markets. For example, to what extent do large fixed supply commitments for future marketings, price rigidities, import or export restrictions, or limited transport and storage capabilities increase the instability of supply in some areas? Could changes in the timing or location of production of particular crops reduce instability? What would be the results of altering combinations of these variables compared to changing the handling of food reserves?

Research should determine if food aid now provided by the major grain exporters and other high-income countries might be reoriented to help the developing countries stabilize their domestic supplies. It has been proposed that the United States, alone or in cooperation with other high-income countries, could guarantee food assistance to the developing countries to compensate for shortfalls in the trend level of annual grain production in excess of a given percentage, such as 6 percent. Such a program should be analyzed to determine its effectiveness on reducing malnutrition, its effects upon the size of reserves held in the developing countries, and its effects upon incentives for farmers and governments to expand food production.

Because food reserves are a worldwide concern, national and international agencies should collaborate on this problem. Alternative ways to manage international cooperation among the national reserve systems should be explored. Suitable research methods include modeling to simulate the effects of alternative policy or program changes on national and international food systems, and comparative analysis of past and current experiments with such changes.

This research must be done largely in cooperation with personnel in the developing countries. International agencies such as FAO, the World Bank, and the International Food Policy Research Institute (IFPRI) can provide leadership and financial and technical inputs. IFPRI is particularly well suited for technical leadership in this field. Research in the United States and in the developing countries should receive financial and technical support from AID and USDA, both of which conduct major programs relevant to this field.

Potential Effects of Research

Food reserves that are an appropriate size and that are managed efficiently could have widespread effects on:

- relieving hunger and malnutrition due to variability of production;
- stabilizing prices and thereby facilitating planning and investment for increased food production;
- encouraging reliance on international trade for a portion of national food supplies;
- expanding direct food distribution to the most deprived groups.

Many developing countries have already taken actions to alter their food systems for the purposes discussed above, and parallel international discussions are underway as a follow-up to the World Food Conference. However, until governments that wish to improve their handling of food reserves are better informed, prospects for satisfactory results will remain poor.

INFORMATION SYSTEMS

Decision makers need timely information to assess the likely effects of alternative decisions. Policies, programs, and research on food and nutrition are becoming more diverse and complex year by year. As the marketing system becomes more complex, information needs increase. In fact, a marketing system provides a great deal of information, but prompt information may also be required from outside of the marketing system. Long-range planning depends on increased information. The use of higher yielding technologies to increase production may inadvertently increase unemployment, balance-of-payments deficits, and social strains. These results may reduce consumer demand and thereby delay any improvement in nutrition. Now that countries depend more on one another for markets and as sources of supply, information systems must include larger geographic areas.

The high-income and the developing countries have many similar information problems and requirements although the developing countries require fewer data and less complex systems. Some developing countries spend sizable portions of their scarce resources on information systems. However, the information is often unused because the data collected are not disseminated or are irrelevant to decision needs.

The proposed research on information systems is often methodological, and hence can be transferred among countries. Experimentation will establish the degree to which these results can be transferred among the United States and the developing nations.

Types of Research

We recommend four lines of research: (1) producer information needs, (2) crop monitoring systems, (3) international data bases for land and nutrition, and (4) total information systems design.

Producer Information Needs The gap between actual and potential use of new technologies in the developing countries exists in part because farmers and others making decisions lack information. Research is needed to identify the kinds of information necessary to encourage use of these technologies. Information needs for different technologies vary but generally include weather predictions and reports, current product price quotations, climatic data, product storage requirements, long-range market outlook, estimates of costs and returns for different levels of input, early warning of disease or pest build-ups, estimates of disease and pest risks, and guidance on the use of inputs.

Research is required on such questions as: what specific data are most important; how can they be acquired on a continuing basis at least cost; how are the data best processed, stored, and recalled; and what kind of equipment and organization will provide the most economical service? Research will have to draw on the experiences of the high-income countries in this area, but should concentrate on the comparative analysis of case studies in the developing countries. It also should include operational experiments when designing information systems that are particularly suited to areas where new technology is being introduced.

Crop Monitoring Systems   An early warning of significant events in worldwide production can improve the decisions made by those involved in food systems, including farmers, consumers, and government managers. The technology to improve global and regional early warning systems is developing rapidly. Such systems may also help to monitor ocean and coastal fisheries keyed to aquatic management. Research should address:

— developing improved yield-estimating models using satellite measurements of meteorological and weather variables such as rainfall, soil moisture, and temperature;
— using remote sensing to measure the radiation characteristics of vegetation in order to assess crop stress and episodic events such as drought, hail, disease, and pestilence;
— developing and using improved sampling and survey techniques, particularly in the developing countries.

Timely and accurate information is needed urgently on a worldwide scale. Current information is inadequate for predicting world food shortages early enough to allow governments to develop remedial policies. Limited experiments show that systems could be developed to assess agricultural resources such as soils, climate and weather, and the production outlook. However, basic and developmental research is required before experimental technologies can be used.

A large part of this research would be conducted within a wider program to develop a statistically sound worldwide sampling and survey for data on food production, food consumption and nutritional value, farm income, income distribution, characteristics of farm firms and rural households, and inputs used in food production. The collection of agricultural data in many developing countries is limited to a few one-time surveys, using an inadequate sample from an outdated list of census respondents. While theoretical principles for sampling are available, more adaptive research is necessary to deal with the unique characteristics of developing countries, the newer computer processing techniques, and the need for systems used in the developing countries to become compatible with a worldwide monitoring system.

International Data Bases for Land and Nutrition Information needs can be met more fully and economically by pooling worldwide information on variables that play a major role in world food production and nutrition. International data bases on land uses and on some aspects of nutrition would be particularly useful. These data bases could enhance the effect of the proposed research in these fields and would result in new methods that could be used for developing other worldwide data bases.

A data base on land uses would combine data on common soil characteristics (such as chemical composition, texture, permeability) with the potential crop performance in each soil under various common environmental circumstances (e.g., moisture, temperature, slope) and farming practices (e.g., fertilization, tillage, and water use practices).

A data base on nutritional impacts would pool data on such factors as sources of nutrients, sources and effects of food contaminants, and the relationship between specific nutrient intakes in common diets and particular types of human performance.

Research is needed on how to design systems that can absorb and integrate a wide variety of data from many sources, that can store it so that it can be recalled quickly and economically, and that can be updated and adjusted to accommodate new research findings and new applications of the data. Such systems should be able to combine and adapt modern data acquisition and storage technologies, such as remote sensing, sampling, and computers, with low-cost data processing and access techniques. This flexibility is necessary for the widespread use of the data base, particularly by the developing countries.

Total Information Systems Design A total information system for any given subject, such as crop production, involves many components. A framework is needed to specify appropriate inputs by disciplines. Ways must be found to deal with equipment, procedure, survey, and statistical design problems. Total systems design also must consider putting together more than one system, possibly across subjects, or across geographic areas. Research at any one time can tackle only the most feasible and urgent parts, but total systems design research looks at the whole. Only this type of research can handle adequately feedback mechanisms, interactive system linkages, collaboration with related areas of interest such as agriculture and space, and the development of information theory.

Research is recommended to:

- Develop a conceptual framework to guide the development of complementary food and nutrition information systems on a global basis. Such a framework should be comprehensive enough not only to accommodate "hardware" and "procedural" questions, but also to address institutional, cultural, and political issues. The framework should facilitate the evaluation of trade-offs between timeliness, accuracy, and relevance of information in decision making.
- Develop new statistical techniques for the collection and analysis of data.
- Identify the technology or procedures necessary to operate the system.

Potential Effects of Research

Improved information systems should result in fewer wrong decisions. The limited information now available on the likely effects of alternative decisions affecting food supply and nutrition, particularly in the developing countries, suggests that such improvement could produce large savings. Not all benefits would be achieved in the short run. Most benefits would be achieved as a result of decades of better-directed development and ongoing social adjustments. In the short run, the main return would arise from a more logical system of thought by which decision makers, from planners to farmers, could approach issues of technological change in agriculture and cultural change in nutrition.

The estimates of unused technology are high—so high, in fact, that the need is increasingly perceived to be to get the research used, not to generate more research. Such perceptions misconstrue the facts, but research on producer information that expands and improves the use of technology could have widespread effects. The effect of development and extension programs rests heavily on the quantity and quality of information provided to farmers and other decision makers in the food supply system, including information from worldwide crop monitoring systems. One important application of the latter kind of information is in the management of food reserves at local, national, and international levels.

3 How To Get the Work Done

The International Framework

The nature and scale of the research agenda identified in Chapter 2, when compared with the extent and location of scientific resources currently available, have led us to three major conclusions, which influence our recommendations for action.

First, a large part of the research needed, especially applied and adaptive research, will have to be carried out in the developing countries, where the most serious shortages of resources for research on food and nutrition exist. Consequently, the capacity of the developing countries for research and its application must be substantially enlarged.

Second, over the last decade a number of international research centers and programs have been established in tropical countries. While these are limited in scope, they have demonstrated important capacities to accomplish research, especially on food production technology in tropical conditions; to reinforce national research organizations in the developing countries; and to build cooperative relationships with scientific groups and centers in North America and Europe. Moreover, international efforts are especially important to the large number of smaller countries that cannot mount large research programs of their own. Consequently, the work of international research centers and programs concerned with food and nutrition should be extended and strengthened.

Third, a large part of the research needed, especially basic research, but also including applied and adaptive research, will have to be done in

North America and Europe where most of the relevant scientific resources are found. We believe that present resources for research on food and nutrition in the United States are seriously inadequate and in important respects inefficiently used. Consequently, the United States should enlarge and reshape its research on food and nutrition.

These three objectives need to be approached in combination, not separately. Building working relationships among research groups in the high-income countries, developing countries, and international centers can bring major benefits to all parties, particularly with respect to nutrition, on which so little research is conducted in any part of the world. (Such collaboration has already begun; see the description of existing international collaboration in rice research in Appendix C.)

All these objectives will require a sustained effort over a period of years, with constant attention to the highest standards of quality. Because we are convinced that the problems of world hunger and malnutrition will be of major importance for at least the next quarter century, we think such an effort is warranted and should be made.

RESEARCH CAPACITY IN THE DEVELOPING COUNTRIES

Most of the increases in food production and improvements in food distribution required to deal with world hunger and malnutrition will need to take place in the developing countries (see Chapter 1). Much of the research required to support those increases and improvements also must be done in those countries.

This is true for technical reasons: the food production and distribution technology that has been devised in North America and Western Europe is largely inappropriate in tropical climates or in the economic circumstances of the developing countries. To design efficient, labor-intensive, and capital-saving techniques for doubling and tripling crop yields in tropical countries, under a great variety of local circumstances, will require research conducted under those conditions. A scientific advance developed elsewhere almost always requires adaptive research in the developing countries before it can be applied. Such research is sometimes highly sophisticated.

As this report has repeatedly emphasized, food production and distribution are social as well as technical processes. Understanding those processes and bringing about changes in them require a sound understanding of the society in question and decisions by its members, including political decisions in many cases. Research on these matters, leading to change, to a large extent has to be done in the countries concerned.

The capacity in the developing countries to conduct research and development on food and nutrition, and to apply the results, is very limited at present. The situation varies substantially among different countries: some, like India or Brazil, have a large and growing scientific community; others have only made a beginning in that direction. But all are far short of the scientific and technical resources they need, as their own scientific leaders are the first to point out. This deficiency is the most serious current impediment to applying research to reduce world hunger and malnutrition.

To meet this deficiency will require a larger and more sustained effort than has been made thus far. The new effort must make the most of the resources available: selecting the most economical methods and facilities; concentrating on the most urgent research problems; using cooperative arrangements under which established researchers in other countries can best contribute to the required work; and using international and regional centers as fully as possible.

Even when all these potential sources of economies are taken into account, there will be substantial need for investment in training researchers and establishing research facilities in the developing countries. We note this realistically, not in discouragement. The prospects are that gains from well-designed research will far exceed the costs.

Where will the resources come from to build research capacity in the developing countries? First and most importantly, they must come from those countries themselves. The recognition by the governments of the developing countries of the importance of research, the commitment of able scientists to the design and management of research organizations, the insistence on standards of local relevance for research institutions, the increased allocation of budgetary resources (including borrowing capacity) to research, the sustained attention to the processes by which research results are actually put to use by those who need them—all these are essential decisions and commitments that can be made only by national leaders and groups within the developing countries.

When such local decisions and commitments are being made, a great deal can be contributed by others. In its meetings with scientific leaders from the developing countries, the Committee asked their views on how the United States could most usefully contribute to the development of research capacity in their countries. Based on their answers, we conclude that:

– The United States should do more—and do it better—to train researchers for the developing countries, both through training indi-

viduals at U.S. universities and through helping build training institutions abroad.
- The United States should do more to aid developing countries in the establishment of research facilities and institutions and in the application of research results.
- The United States should do more to encourage and support communication and collaboration among researchers in the developing countries, in international and regional institutions, and in the United States, on problems of common interest.

The recommendations presented later in this chapter address all these objectives.

A word should be said about the likely evolution of research relevant to the developing countries. There is a natural division of labor at present, with the heaviest load of applied and adaptive research falling on researchers (whatever their nationality) working in the developing countries, and the heaviest load of fundamental research falling on researchers (whatever their nationality) working in the high-income countries. Even now the division is not absolute; there are capable scientists in the developing countries working productively on fundamental problems. Over time, with the growth of scientific communities and research capacity in the developing countries, larger amounts of fundamental research will be conducted there. The important point from the standpoint of the United States is that if our scientific communities concerned with food and nutrition develop and maintain effective international associations, the United States can only gain from the evolution. Already, for example, U.S. agriculture has benefited greatly from research conducted at the International Maize and Wheat Improvement Center (CIMMYT) in Mexico.

INTERNATIONAL RESEARCH CENTERS AND PROGRAMS

Perhaps the largest research contributions to increasing the world supply of food in recent years have been made by the international agricultural research centers, especially CIMMYT and the International Rice Research Institute in the Philippines. These centers have achieved important research results, such as developing the semidwarf varieties of wheat and rice; they have become important training locations; and they have contributed to the enlargement of research capacity in a number of developing countries.

It is important not to exaggerate the potential significance of international research centers and programs. They cannot substitute, for example, for the careful, detailed, location-specific activities needed to adapt high yielding varieties to local circumstances. Nor can they substitute for the diverse, extensive attempt to advance fundamental knowledge that takes place primarily in universities.

In their limited sphere, however, international centers and programs have a powerful potential, and they need to be continued and strengthened. Financing is currently provided for the principal centers by members of the Consultative Group on International Agricultural Research (CGIAR: a coordinating committee of donor organizations, including agencies of national governments, foundations, and international organizations, jointly sponsored by the World Bank, FAO, and the U.N. Development Program). Total funding is about $80 million per year, of which about 25 percent is provided by the U.S. government. A recent careful review by CGIAR suggests that these costs should rise to $120 million by 1980.

There are a number of international research centers and programs not sponsored by CGIAR that are relevant to world hunger and malnutrition. For example, a complex but effective institution is the Global Atmospheric Research Program which welds the strength of an intergovernmental organization, the World Meteorological Organization, to that of an international nongovernmental scientific organization, the International Council of Scientific Unions, in the interest of coordinating worldwide climate research.

We conclude that:

– The United States should continue to provide 25 percent of the funding for the centers and programs sponsored by CGIAR.
– The United States also should join in supporting other high quality international centers and programs, both those it is already involved with and others for which it is not now a major supporter.
– In addition, the United States should move vigorously and imaginatively to encourage collaborative relationships between international centers and research groups in the United States.

Our recommendations, later in this chapter, address these objectives.

U.S. RESEARCH ON FOOD AND NUTRITION

The Committee believes U.S. research on food and nutrition should serve two main purposes: (1) it should enable future U.S. food production and distribution to meet domestic needs at reasonable prices while permitting the continued export of major amounts of food; and (2) it should help to increase food production and improve food distribution in the developing countries. Considered against these purposes, and in light of the research agenda presented in Chapter 2, we are convinced that the current U.S. research capacity needs substantial enlargement and reshaping. Specifically, we conclude that:

- Major increases are needed in fundamental research, both in the natural and in the social sciences, related to the enhancement of food production and nutrition; this will require stepped-up training of the necessary researchers, some new facilities, and mobilization of scientific resources not previously involved.
- A new and broader approach is needed for research on nutrition. More epidemiologic studies are needed on the interrelations of nutrition and human development, nutrition and disease, nutrition and productivity. Nutrition research should be more closely related to the rest of the food system and its institutional components, from production through marketing to consumption.
- The U.S. research community should give much greater attention to international objectives. Much of the research done in the United States, particularly toward the fundamental end of the research spectrum, can serve users both in the United States and in the developing countries, if priorities are set and results communicated with overseas users in mind. Some U.S. research will need to be directed specifically to the problems of the developing countries; such research will require special arrangements for international training and support for U.S. researchers. In our view, these changes will not only permit the United States to contribute to the reduction of world hunger and malnutrition, but also will permit the United States to obtain greater benefits from international scientific collaboration.
- Support for social science research relevant to food and nutrition problems should be increased sharply. We were impressed in the course of our study by the inadequacy of the policy analysis being used in the United States as well as in other countries to address questions about food and nutrition, and the correspondingly urgent need for the underlying social science research needed to support better analysis. In addition, social science research is needed to help determine priorities for production research, to measure the effects of technological change, to improve the functioning of markets and other institutional arrangements serving rural development, and for many other purposes.

Recommendations for U.S. Action

THE FEDERAL–STATE SYSTEM OF AGRICULTURAL RESEARCH

Our first set of recommendations concerns the federal–state agricultural research system, and the role of the Department of Agriculture. We make several recommendations calling for a substantial increase in the scale of and a substantial reorientation in the content and objectives of U.S. agricultural research.

We consider these recommendations to be the most important we are making on organization and financing. They are intended to enable the Department of Agriculture, in cooperation with the state experiment stations and other universities and private research groups, to make a much larger contribution to reducing world hunger and malnutrition than it has thus far.

If our recommendations are to become effective, the Department of Agriculture, the state experiment stations, and others involved in agricultural research will need to put much more emphasis on fundamental research (without reducing their concern for applied research). They will need to mobilize scientific resources from universities and parts of universities that have not previously been involved with agricultural research. They will need to design new and broader approaches to nutrition, and give greater emphasis to the social sciences. They will need to add to their traditional focus on the United States a direct and explicit concern with hunger and malnutrition overseas, especially in the developing countries. And they will need to carry forward these efforts on a sustained basis over at least the next two decades.

We believe the time is ripe for these changes, and that those concerned with agricultural research and the uses of its results will agree that these alterations are overdue.

• *We recommend the appointment of an Assistant Secretary of Agriculture with responsibility only for research and education.*

Whether this is accomplished by realignment of existing responsibilities or by establishing a new post is immaterial. The important points are:

– To accomplish changes of the extent and nature that are required, a single senior officer, reporting directly to the Secretary, should be made responsible for the major research and educational programs of the department.

- The Assistant Secretary should be a senior scientist or scientific administrator of sufficient stature to make plain the seriousness with which the President and the Secretary are approaching food and nutrition research and to attract the highest quality scientific advisers and participants outside as well as inside the traditional agricultural research establishment.
- The Assistant Secretary should be given supervision over the Agricultural Research Service, the Cooperative State Research Service (CSRS), the Economic Research Service (ERS), the Statistical Reporting Service, the Extension Service, the National Agricultural Library, and the new agency we are recommending to administer a competitive grants program.
- The Assistant Secretary should be given specific mandates to establish a major program of support for research on nutrition in the department, and to develop strong international dimensions within the several research programs under his or her direction.

A special word should be said about the Economic Research Service, which now performs important policy advisory and assessment functions for the Secretary in addition to its research role. We believe the Secretary needs, directly available to him, a strong policy advisory and assessment unit. We also believe that the role of the social sciences in agricultural research needs to be substantially enhanced, and that one major step in that direction would be to transfer ERS, less its policy advisory and assessment functions, to join the cluster of research agencies under the Assistant Secretary. Furthermore, ERS should be given a significantly stronger staff, with competence not only in economics but in the other social sciences as well. Relating social science research and agricultural production research more closely could make each of them more effective.

- *We recommend substantial increases in federal funding for the traditional* USDA *research programs (including support for state programs), and we recommend funds to establish a new program of competitive grants for research on food and nutrition.*

Increased funding through traditional channels will provide new vitality for the existing system. Competitive grants will be a principal means of increasing support for fundamental research, for drawing on scientific resources outside the traditional agricultural research establishment, and for new and broader research efforts concerned with nutrition. These two strands of increased funding will be complementary: the outcome of each will permit stronger results from the other. Both elements should develop the increased international orientation stressed above. Both will support accelerated research in the priority areas recommended in Chapter 2.

• *We recommend a first-year increase on the order of $120 million, something under 20 percent of the total of about $700 million of* USDA *and state funds now devoted to food and nutrition research. We propose that the new funds be divided equally between the existing federal–state channels and the new competitive grants program. Thereafter, we recommend successive increases, after adjustments for inflation, on the order of $60 million or approximately 10 percent per year in real terms for the next four years, also divided evenly between the existing programs and the new competitive grants program.*

These proposed increases should be reviewed annually and revised as experience may suggest. Longer term funding plans should be based on a thorough review of the situation and outlook toward the end of this five-year period.

We think it appropriate that these funds come from the federal government, since their purposes are largely national and international in character. At the same time, we expect that they should and will attract substantial additional funds from the states, since they will benefit from improvements in U.S. production.

There is no doubt that funding increases on this scale or larger are needed, not only to undertake the large research agenda identified in Chapter 2, but also to overcome the effects of the relative neglect of agricultural research in recent decades when more glamorous subjects like health and space preempted a large portion of new funds and talent. At the same time, we have endorsed a conservative rate of build-up with the conviction that continuity, stability, and steady growth are vital to the planning of effective research programs.

Three points are worthy of special note. First, a substantial share of the increased funds will be needed to expand the U.S. personnel base, both by educating young researchers and encouraging career shifts by established investigators. There are many researchers now employed in other fields who are capable of significant contributions to food and nutrition research if they can be attracted to this field, either as full-time investigators or through part-time involvement in interdisciplinary efforts. Not only do we need more scientists working on food and nutrition, but more scientists with experience and understanding of conditions in other parts of the world. A systematic effort will be needed under both the federal–state programs and the competitive grants program to achieve these objectives.

Second, we urge that a major new emphasis be placed on nutritional research by the Department of Agriculture. Such research should, of course, not duplicate that carried out by NIH; as we note below, we believe the NIH research should be continued and strengthened. The Department of Agriculture should focus on the relationships between nutrition and the food system from production through delivery, on the possibilities and effects of nutritional programs, and on the desirability of alternative nutritional policies—questions that have been largely ignored in the United States as in other countries, and with respect to which the United States has much to gain from participating in international collaborative research.

Third, we emphasize the importance of establishing a strong competitive grants program in the Department of Agriculture. The program should draw on the best experience of other agencies that have administered competitive grants. Eligibility should be open to all comers, from the public and private sectors, and awards should be based on peer review. Strong advisory committees should be established including natural and social scientists of outstanding ability who could encourage able colleagues to become interested in these fields. Predoctoral and postdoctoral fellowships should be available. The main instrument for research support should be renewable project grants, of three years' duration, although institutional grants for minimal operating expenses may be warranted in some cases, particularly where international knowledge and relationships need to be built up and maintained.

The competitive grants program in food and nutrition should experiment with ways to encompass international concerns: for example, foreign scientists might be included on advisory committees and review panels to make sure that international as well as U.S. interests are appropriately considered; predoctoral and postdoctoral research awards might be provided at appropriate national and international research centers abroad as well as in the United States. Imaginative, multidisciplinary approaches to problems of global importance should be encouraged.

In the administration of the program, we think the operating principles just outlined will be more important than the organizational framework. We recognize that the 1978 budget submitted to Congress contains $27.6 million for a competitive grants program of the type we are recommending, although more limited in scope, which would be administered within CSRS. We applaud this recognition of the need for such a program. At the same time, we would suggest that consideration be given to administering the program through a separate agency or office reporting directly to the Assistant Secretary. A program of the scale and complexity we are proposing, heavily oriented toward fundamental research, would pose problems of management sufficiently different from the traditional functions of CSRS to argue for independent administration.

• *We recommend a five-year federal matching grants program for nonfederal research facilities and equipment. These grants should be available to other universities and private nonprofit institutions as well as those in the land-grant group.*

The rationale for this program is twofold. First, large additional resources are needed for altering and replacing existing facilities, which have had very little improvement over the past decade and are in many cases cramped and obsolete. Second, additional facilities will be needed to carry out the research agenda we have developed, including a few wholly new installations such as special containment facilities for research involving recombinant DNA; one or more centers for collecting, evaluating, distributing, and doing applied research on nitrogen-fixing bacteria; and one or more strong tropical research centers in the United States.

The Committee did not have much data on which to base a judgment about the appropriate scale for a facilities funding program. Such information as we had, however, suggests that federal funds as large as $100 million per year might be well and prudently used. Our assumption is that, in the normal case, the federal funds for particular facilities would be matched equally by nonfederal funds, although in a few cases the national or international purposes of the facility may suggest a federal share larger than 50 percent of the cost.

In addition to the requirements for upgrading nonfederal research facilities and equipment, we believe there is also some need within the federal research establishment for modernization, replacement of obsolete equipment, and some new facilities designed for new tasks.

These recommendations—for establishing stronger research leadership in the Department of Agriculture, and for enlarging substantially the funding available for research support and facilities, including the establishment of a major competitive grants program—constitute our major recommendations for the Department's role in accomplishing the research and development tasks outlined in Chapter 2. They constitute a large and demanding set of tasks and changes in the Department's traditional ways of doing things. A major effort, ably led and sustained over a number of years, will be required if our recommendations are to become effective.

Before leaving the role of the Department of Agriculture, it is important to reemphasize that, to carry out these recommendations, USDA and the state experiment stations—and the legislators who vote their authority and funds—must take a different approach toward international problems than they have in the past. We do not suggest that department funds be used to support the establishment or operation of national research organizations in other countries; to the extent that U.S. funds are properly used for such purposes, we consider the Agency for International Development the appropriate administering agency. But we do believe it necessary that Department of Agriculture funds be used to enable the U.S. scientific community concerned with food and nutrition to become involved in international efforts: to join in collaborative research with colleagues abroad, to conduct research in overseas locations, to undertake training and postdoctoral fellowships in research centers abroad, and to invite foreign scientists to work at U.S. research facilities for limited periods. More than funding is involved; USDA and the universities will need to modify the reward system for professional work so that international experience will hasten advancement and generate special recognition.

The United States has a major and growing stake in such international research collaboration with other high-income countries as well as with the developing countries. The Department of Agriculture already sends teams abroad for specific purposes, such as studying animal diseases that are or could become important in the United States. Substantial enlargement of such international research collaboration is needed and should be supported by specific legislative mandates based on the recognition that the United States has much to gain, as well as much to give. For example, more work is being done currently in countries other than the United States on biological nitrogen fixation and on genetic work at the cell level in plants, and U.S. scientists could gain results of immediate benefit to our country if they participated in research on nutrition in the developing countries.

This conception of USDA's role in international research is consistent with a broad view of its concern for world food and nutrition. It has sometimes been thought that USDA should reflect primarily the commercial concerns of U.S. agricultural producers. Those interests are important, and entitled to appropriate weight in the international policies of the United States. But as a nation we have other important interests as well: helping to lessen the hunger of half the world, and encouraging economic and social progress as an essential element in world peace and order. In our view, the Secretary of Agriculture speaks not just for the interest of American food producers but also for the broader interests of all American citizens in a world moving to alleviate hunger and malnutrition. During a period in which it appears likely that the world will remain on the verge of major food shortages, the chance of serious conflict between the narrower and broader interests seems small. Nevertheless, we should be explicit about the principles involved.

AGENCY FOR INTERNATIONAL DEVELOPMENT

AID is the natural vehicle for stronger U.S. action to help establish research and development capacity in the developing countries, to support further development of international research centers and programs, and to support the involvement of U.S. scientific groups in research concerned with food and nutrition in the developing countries. Our recommendations propose substantial increases in the scale of and improvements in the substance of AID's activities to these ends. Title XII of the Foreign Assistance Act, enacted in late 1975, provides a new and much stronger legislative base for these activities, and for the participation of U.S. universities in them. We shall discuss this further.

At the outset, however, we note a major concern. Over recent years, owing to the effects of staffing reductions, the customary legislative uncertainty, and other factors, AID has suffered a serious depletion of its professional staff concerned with agriculture and with science more broadly. If AID is to play the strong role we envision in taking advantage of the opportunities opened by Title XII, and in cooperating effectively with USDA, NSF, NIH, and other government agencies concerned with research, it must rebuild its past competence and in important respects add expert knowledge it has lacked. The large resources of the universities and other U.S. entities cannot be mobilized and applied to the needs of the developing countries unless there is a high quality professional cadre in AID. Their number need not be great, but the building of such a cadre should be a top priority for AID in the immediate future.

• *We recommend a larger and more systematic effort by* AID *to help the developing countries establish research and development capabilities for food and nutrition in both the natural and social sciences.*

As with other types of development assistance, outside help can only be effective where local commitment, energy, and resources are present. Given those conditions, AID can mobilize public and private resources to help in several ways: with the design of appropriate research programs, facilities, and organizations; with initial advisory consulting and staffing services; with training for research and technical staff members; and with contributions toward research costs.

Designing and building research organizations that will influence the actual course of food production and consumption in the varied historical and cultural settings of different countries is very difficult. Persistence and intelligence are more important than large sums of money at the outset. The risks are great that copies of American agricultural research stations and social science research centers will be set up and, while well staffed and well equipped, will not be effectively related to local problems, policymakers, and action organizations.

Although these elements present serious problems, the objective remains essential and AID, supported by Congress, should make a strong and enduring commitment to it. The scale of funds needed would not be great compared to the potential benefits. AID expenditures in this category have been rising and recently are running at about $30 million per year. In our view, that figure should be at least tripled by the early 1980s. In planning the future scale of U.S. assistance for this purpose, AID should recognize the increasing interest of the World Bank and other bilateral aid donors, and work with them in assisting the development of research capabilities in the developing countries.

• *We recommend a larger and better-designed* AID *effort to train research personnel for the developing countries.*

Such an effort should have two main components. The first involves work with U.S. universities to improve the quality and relevance of their training for foreign students. Relatively large numbers of such students are educated in the United States, financed by a wide variety of sources including public and private agencies in the United States, international agencies, and public and private sources in the students' home countries. But there has been relatively little effort to develop specialized programs that could make their education more relevant, nor do the universities have enough staff members with the experience and knowledge necessary to advise students on conducting research in their home countries. The universities themselves, working with AID, have a major responsibility to improve this situation.

The second part of the effort involves helping to establish research training programs in the developing countries themselves. Most research personnel will be trained at home, partly on the job and partly in academic settings, although smaller numbers of research leaders needing education at the doctoral or postdoctoral levels will have to obtain it in the United States or other high-income countries for some years to come. To help establish effective research training programs, including special attention to the needs of research educators, administrators, and managers, should be a distinct and important part of AID's work.

In the process of improving research training in the developing countries, in the United States, and in the international centers, new methods to develop tyeps of international cooperation that combine strong academic work with field research in the developing countries should be encouraged.

• *We recommend the establishment of a joint* AID–*university committee on international training under Title XII of the Foreign Assistance Act.*

Several aspects of research training require close cooperation between AID and U.S. universities. The proposed committee could give prominence and leadership to the training aspect of building research capabilities in the developing countries, an aspect that has too long been underemphasized.

• *We recommend continuation of* AID *support for international research centers and programs, both those supported by the Consultative Group on International Agricultural Research and others of worldwide or regional scope that are likely to provide research results that are badly needed by the developing countries.*

There are special risks in establishing international or regional research centers, which can be remote from reality and from desirable pressures to make a substantial difference in the world. But there are also special opportunities for concentration of high quality talent on significant subjects, with unusual freedom from political and other extraneous influences. International centers can contribute significantly to the build-up of research capacity in the developing countries. They can work as partners with institutions in high-income countries, linking those who work on more applied with those that work on more fundamental research problems.

To achieve the potential advantages and avoid the pitfalls, it is desirable to limit such centers and programs to those few that are clearly of unusual promise, to organize them in such a way as to ensure the highest quality scientific management and staffing, and to assure their working relationships with research centers in the developing and high-income countries. When these conditions are met, such centers and programs can be highly productive.

This is clearly the case thus far with respect to the centers supported by CGIAR; U.S. contributions to those centers, which amount to about $20 million per year at present and are scheduled to rise by about $4 million per year over the next several years, are clearly money well spent. U.S. contributions are based on a 25 percent formula, which has had a stabilizing effect on the overall financial support system of the CGIAR centers and has encouraged support from other quarters.

We have not tried to review all the other international centers and programs to which the United States might usefully contribute. We note, however, the value of the International Fertilizer Development Center in Alabama which draws on the experience of the Tennessee Valley Authority, and of the International Soybean Program in Illinois, which draws on the special knowledge of the University of Illinois and the USDA soybean laboratory. While both are located in the United States, their principal purpose is to respond to problems of the developing nations, and it is therefore appropriate that U.S. contributions to their costs be provided through AID. We note also the special case of the Asian Vegetable Research and Development Center in Taiwan, to which the United States contributes substantially. Additional centers to which the United States might consider contributing include the International Center for Insect Physiology and Ecology in Kenya, the International Center for Living Aquatic Resources Management in the Philippines, and some of the nutrition centers that are becoming international resources under the initial programs of the United Nations University.

International research centers and programs are a relatively new phenomenon and many complex issues will arise in deciding when to establish, enlarge, and terminate them, how to achieve and sustain high quality performance in them, and what the United States can and should contribute to them. One important set of questions concerns the best way to strengthen research on production factors that affect commodities generally (e.g., work on water or insects) and relate such research to research on individual commodities (e.g., work on rice or cassava). It might be helpful for AID to establish a small advisory committee, including scientists from government and private organizations, to help deal with these questions. The promise of such international efforts is high and worth major attention.

• *We recommend that* AID *enlarge significantly its support for establishing operating relationships between U.S. research groups and those in the developing countries.*

With the winding down of an earlier generation of institution-building projects, the U.S. universities' knowledge of conditions in the developing countries, and their direct involvement in those countries, have been declining. A number of actions are needed to reverse this trend, and many of them can and should be supported by AID under Title XII.

We commend the concept, now being developed under Title XII, of support for multiyear research programs—planned for at least five years—linking U.S. and overseas researchers interested in a common scientific field or problem, such as adapting soybean cultivation to tropical conditions, or management of tropical soils, or relationships between diet patterns and human performance, or expanding the use of coastal zone aquaculture. Such programs should serve simultaneously to advance knowledge, train young scientists from the developing countries and from the United States for work on problems of the developing countries, and establish experience and performance standards for research in those countries. This pattern should be expanded to significant areas of social science research, particularly those involving comparative analysis of experience in different places. AID and the Congress must recognize that continuity of support for such programs is essential to their success.

Other forms of support also should be considered. For example, it might be wise for AID to offer to share the cost of some minimum commitment of staff time and support services with any university or research center wishing to establish a serious continuing interest in research in the developing countries. The costs of such arrangements would be small but the potential benefits might be large.

We emphasize that AID, while concerned mainly with the poorest countries, should not hesitate to support research connections with middle-income countries such as Brazil or Mexico. Such countries offer some of the best opportunities for valuable and relatively inexpensive exchanges of research collaboration. These opportunities stem in part from previous AID investments. AID has authority to support international research collaboration wherever it advances program goals such as improving the world food situation, and should use this authority vigorously.

We also emphasize that Title XII activities should strengthen nutrition work in AID and university programs, putting greater stress on investigations of the effects of diet patterns on human functional performance, and on the effects on nutrition of governmental policies concerning agriculture, food distribution, and development in general.

Finally, we note the critical threshold on which AID, the universities—both land-grant universities and others—and the Department of Agriculture stand as the implementation of Title XII begins. Significant improvements are needed in AID's staffing and in its traditional procedures in order to provide support on a continuing basis for good university planning and management of international research. The universities need to make a commitment to sustained international work and to recognize that, while they will benefit by gaining experience for their own research and teaching functions, the aim of Title XII is to help the developing countries primarily by supporting work there. USDA needs to lend its strength to the AID–university collaboration in many ways, and AID–USDA collaboration needs to be greatly strengthened. There are encouraging signs that all the parties recognize these needs, but much work lies ahead to meet them.

NATIONAL INSTITUTES OF HEALTH

NIH is the largest source of federal support for research on human nutrition, spending about $60 million per year. Most of this research is oriented to the interrelationships between diets and diseases prevalent in the United States.

• *We recommend that NIH's support for nutrition research be reoriented to place greater emphasis on studies of human subjects, particularly using epidemiologic approaches and behavioral and other social science skills.*

It is time for NIH to reach out for a broader range of scientific talent to become involved in nutrition research, and to seek new and fresh approaches to the subject. Because the necessary skills are scarce, support for training programs as well as research will be required.

• *We recommend that more effective arrangements be established for coordinating research on nutrition supported by the several Institutes and by other relevant agencies in the Department of Health, Education, and Welfare.*

A dozen NIH Institutes and the Food and Drug Administration are involved in nutrition research, while numerous other parts of the Department of Health, Education, and Welfare operate nutrition programs. Each agency has tended to approach the subject autonomously, although their programs have many overlapping concerns.

We believe there is a natural division of labor between research on human nutrition supported by NIH and that which would, under our recommendations, be supported through the Department of Agriculture.

The NIH-supported research would begin with biological factors and the relationships between nutrition and human behavior, and nutrition and disease, and would reach out toward the social settings in which people obtain and use food. The USDA-supported research would begin with the systems of food production and distribution, and with the effect and usefulness of program interventions, and would reach out toward biological and health issues. In setting research priorities, both groups should pay great attention to nutritional conditions in the developing countries. Much of what everyone needs to know can be learned there.

• *We recommend only modest increments in the NIH budget for nutrition research for the immediate future. Some funds from lower priority programs should be diverted to higher priority purposes. In the longer run, we have no doubt that larger funds will be required.*

NATIONAL SCIENCE FOUNDATION

The central mission of the National Science Foundation is to nurture the health of the science disciplines and their output of basic knowledge by grants for fundamental disciplinary research and training. Support for basic work in the plant sciences and for other science activities that could contribute to food and nutrition concerns is relatively modest— about $40 million or 5 percent of the fiscal year 1977 NSF program budget. Support for basic work in the social sciences is only about $20 million. Large and sustained increases are needed in these sums in order to enlarge as rapidly as possible the stock of fundamental knowledge on which future applied research will depend.

• *We recommend that the National Science Foundation substantially increase its support of fundamental research in biology and other natural science disciplines underlying work on food and nutrition.*

Considering the volume of high quality research applications not now being funded, we believe present support levels could be doubled within three years, with further expansion thereafter depending on the quality of applications.

• *We also recommend strengthened support by NSF for disciplinary research in the social and behavioral sciences relevant to food and nutrition.*

• *We recommend that funding increases be complemented by increasing the size and duration of individual project financing.*

Projects have averaged about $38,000 per year and most grants are for two years. Such limitations have sometimes precluded important research and have created inefficient ratios of administrative costs to direct research costs. NSF should accelerate progress on major research problems, particularly in the early stages of the work, by encouraging patterns of individual research grants that are mutually reinforcing and by providing for periodic workshops or other systematic consultation among the grantees.

Any tendency to discourage basic research applications in which crops or animals are the subjects should be eliminated. Under the recommendations we are making, mission-oriented basic research funded through the Department of Agriculture will naturally address fundamental questions as they arise, and will include such fields as plant physiology and plant cell biology, in which NSF should also be working. Possible overlaps of this kind are not a matter for concern if there is good coordination. The only danger is that significant gaps will appear in the research coverage as has happened in the past.

The authorizing legislation for NSF for fiscal year 1977 places special emphasis on international scientific collaboration to assist in resolving critical world problems such as those of food and population.

• *We recommend vigorous action by* NSF *under this new mandate to promote international scientific collaboration.*

Particularly with respect to the developing countries, such joint efforts can enlarge research capacity while producing important research results. One way to build science research capability in the developing countries, for example, is to provide grants for U.S. scientists to work for limited periods with colleagues in those countries on research or teaching programs. It is particularly useful to enable outstanding postdoctoral research fellows to stay overseas for, say, one to three years. The U.S.–Brazil chemistry program developed by the National Academy of Sciences is a good example of this approach. NSF, under its new mandate, is a logical source of support for such efforts.

The fiscal year 1977 authorizing legislation also puts new stress on training in interdisciplinary research, including research grants.

• *We recommend that a program of training in interdisciplinary research be undertaken because of its potential for dealing with food and nutrition problems.*

At the same time, successful experience with interdisciplinary research is rare, and we suggest that NSF support efforts to understand the conditions for success in such research—alternative methodologies, institutional frameworks, types of research training, and other factors.

OTHER GOVERNMENT AGENCIES

Other U.S. government agencies conduct or regulate research and development relating to food and nutrition. This includes work by the Environmental Protection Agency, the Energy Research and Development Administration, and the Department of the Interior on the use of resources going into agriculture; research affecting food processing and marketing by the Departments of Transportation, Commerce, Defense, and Health, Education, and Welfare; weather and fisheries research by several agencies; and policy research by still other agencies on issues affecting world trade, U.S. access to world resources, and other relevant concerns. (See Appendix D for a fuller account.) We have not made recommendations concerning each agency because of the detailed consideration that would have been necessary. We believe, nevertheless, that these recommendations are important and should be developed, and this is one of the reasons we consider it essential to establish a continuous monitoring and leadership organization in the Executive Office of the President, as recommended later.

PRIVATELY SUPPORTED RESEARCH

Currently, roughly half of U.S. research and development concerned with food and nutrition is financed in the private sector. While a small fraction of this is provided by nonprofit organizations, the great bulk is from business firms representing a wide range of industrial pursuits: food processing and distribution; agricultural inputs such as fertilizer, seed, feed, and farm machinery; food and nutrition-related drugs and chemicals; and many more.

The research and development activities of these firms are chiefly concerned with product development; even when more basic research is involved there is usually a product-oriented objective. Business decisions on the scale and priorities of research and development activities are, naturally, primarily influenced by considerations of potential sales and markets.

Over time a rough but effective division of labor has emerged, with government-financed research and development tending to be the scientific end of the spectrum and business-financed research tending toward development of products. The two have been complementary in important ways.

The question relevant to this report is what action can or should be taken to enable privately financed research and development to contribute more to alleviate world food and nutrition problems in the years ahead. The Committee was able to study only limited aspects of the question, and reached the following conclusions.

• *We recommend that* AID *enlarge its use of contracts to draw on the capacity of private companies to contribute to research and research training objectives in the developing countries.*

Such arrangements must be carefully worked out to ensure that all parties understand and agree on the work to be done, and to ensure that end results benefit local research personnel and institutions in the developing countries. But the potential benefits, particularly teaching the skills of translating research knowledge into production practices and of motivating producers to try something new, are sufficiently large to warrant the effort. For example, in fields such as food preservation, processing, and packaging, the resources in the U.S. private sector ought to be capable of major contributions.

• *We also recommend that the Department of Agriculture consider the possibility of making greater use of private resources, by contract, for needed aspects of food and nutrition research where that may bring effective results at equal or smaller public cost.*

Another possibility for exploration is shared public and private financing of product development research in cases in which the product market is not adequate to attract full-cost financing by private firms.

Two factors potentially inhibiting the usefulness of normal, market-oriented research and development by private business should be noted. The first is the possibility that government regulations established in the interest of health, safety, environmental protection, and other purposes may through overlapping, imprecision, or other effects create unnecessary or unwise limitations on research and development. The subject is immensely complex and applies to many fields, but we consider it a serious problem in connection with food and nutrition.

• *We recommend that coordination and simplification of regulations affecting research and development on food and nutrition be given early attention.*

This is best done under the leadership of the Executive Office of the President, using arrangements recommended in the next section.

A second set of problems involves patent rights. Issues being raised in international forums and the actions being taken by a number of foreign governments challenge the validity, and therefore the effectiveness, of patents and proprietary rights. Questions about the adequacy of U.S. patent laws, as these apply to research on plants, also may be posed by the current and prospective broadening of techniques of genetic manipulation. Patent protection is a very complex subject that affects companies in many other fields as well as food and nutrition.

   • *We recommend an early evaluation of U.S. and international proprietary rights under the leadership of the Executive Office of the President.*

EXECUTIVE OFFICE OF THE PRESIDENT

The preceding pages amply illustrate the complexity of the task the President identified in his letter to the National Academy of Sciences: to enable U.S. research and development capacity to play a more powerful part in alleviating world hunger and malnutrition. From the beginning of its deliberations, the Committee repeatedly addressed the question of how to achieve coherence among the many different actions that need to be taken and the many governmental and private agencies that are necessarily involved. We reached two central conclusions with which Study Team 14 concurred:

– It is necessary to establish in the Executive Office of the President arrangements for designing and implementing a coherent strategy for research on food and nutrition.
– Such a research strategy can be established only within the framework of a coherent general strategy for dealing with world food and nutrition problems, which also requires Executive Office leadership.

In reaching these conclusions, we have explicitly rejected the notion of strong central control through some sort of super-bureaucracy. What we have in mind is quite different. We think operational authority, funds, and programs should be retained in the various departments and agencies. At the same time, a central capacity is needed to look well ahead at overall problems, to organize a common basis of understanding and analysis among the different operational programs, to assess the overall effectiveness of U.S. policies and programs, and to raise issues concerning coherence and effectiveness for joint consideration or, if necessary, presidential decision.

There are various organizational alternatives for achieving these ends: an interdepartmental group with a small staff, a Cabinet subcommittee with a small staff, or a special council with a small staff. The essential characteristics are capable leadership and an independent staff. We have not felt it necessary to express a preference among these alternatives, especially at this time when a new administration is developing its own patterns for responding to requirements of this kind.

However, we do insist that certain needs be served. First, with respect to the general strategy for dealing with world food and nutrition problems, there must be an Executive Office entity that can look simultaneously at: domestic and foreign needs for food; alternative policies involving U.S. trade, production, transport, storage, and distribution of food and commodities used to produce food; U.S. commercial and noncommercial interests in world food and nutrition needs; environmental and energy questions in relation to food; and so on. Second, with respect to research strategy, there must be an Executive Office entity (which might be linked both to the food and nutrition policy entity just described and to the Office of Science and Technology Policy), that can monitor and assess the research activities of the several federal agencies involved and the interrelationships between the United States and worldwide research communities.

• *We recommend the establishment of these two entities in the Executive Office of the President: one to develop and maintain a coherent U.S. strategy for dealing with world food and nutrition problems; the other, subordinate to the first, to facilitate coordination of U.S. and international research activities on food and nutrition.*

We came to these recommendations only after considering and rejecting three other alternatives. One would be to draw all sizable federal involvements in food and nutrition into a single agency, a broadened USDA, thereby eliminating most of the requirements for interdepartmental coordination. The difficulty with this is that the functions of the major agencies that affect U.S. involvements in world food and nutrition problems are too integral to their basic responsibilities to be pulled out and amalgamated in a single agency. It is not feasible, for example, to remove major concerns for policies on food trade from the general concern for foreign trade of the Departments of State, Commerce, and the Treasury; or to remove concern for diet–disease relationships from NIH; or to remove concern for agricultural developments in developing countries from the general concern for international development of AID; or to remove concern for energy uses in food production from the general concern with energy uses of the government's energy agencies. There are many more illustrations but the conclusion is clear: a substantial number of federal agencies inevitably are concerned with U.S. policies and actions affecting food and nutrition, and some sort of coordinating arrangement is necessary to achieve coherence among them.

The second alternative would be to make the Secretary of Agriculture responsible for the coordinating functions. He would chair and his department would provide staff for an interagency committee established for this purpose. This pattern, giving one department the "lead agency" role, has been tried in various forms in the past. The evidence suggests that an interagency committee of this type could be useful as an advisory service to USDA, but would not be an effective means of achieving harmonization of the situation appraisals and strategic planning of the many agencies concerned with U.S. and world food problems. Other agencies are not willing to submit their most strongly felt interests to a committee chaired and staffed by USDA. They will do so only in a situation in which they can meet as equals, under higher authority that demands effective coordination, and are served by strong staff work independent of the special interests that inevitably bear on the line agencies.

The small unit in the Executive Office of the President, if strongly led, can meet these requirements for effectiveness. Moreover, from that location, it can work effectively with other elements of the Executive Office such as the Office of Management and Budget, the Council of Economic Advisers, the Office of Science and Technology Policy, and the National Security Council. It can borrow staff specialists from these offices to help with its analytical work, and can provide to those offices appraisals of food and nutrition issues that reflect a governmental overview. We believe also that such a unit would give the USDA a better opportunity than would the "lead agency" concept to influence the operations of other agencies that affect USDA's concerns.

The third alternative would be to establish only a research coordinating unit in the Office of Science and Technology Policy, without a broader unit for coordinating food and nutrition policies. The difficulty with this is that sensible research policies can be established only within a broader framework of U.S. policies concerning food and nutrition. For example, for reasons related in Chapter 1, we think most of the increased food needed in the developing countries over the rest of the century should be produced in those countries, and our recommendations for research reflect that conclusion. But it would make no sense for U.S. government policies concerning food research to move in this direction if other U.S. government policies, regarding, say, the export of fertilizer or world trade in food, were moving in other directions. Consequently, we see no acceptable alternative to the conclusion that there ought to be in the Executive Office of the President both an arrangement for achieving a coherent strategy for research on food and nutrition and an arrangement for achieving a coherent general strategy toward world food and nutrition problems.

A   *Tables*

TABLE 1   Annual grain consumption (actual and projected), by main types of uses, 1970-1990

	Actual consumption	Projected demand*		
	1970	1980	1985	1990
Developed countries				
		(million tons)		
Food	160.9	163.1	164.1	164.6
Feed	371.5	467.9	522.7	565.7
Other uses	84.9	100.6	109.5	116.4
TOTAL	617.3	731.6	796.3	846.7
		(kilograms)		
Per capita	576	623	649	663
Developing market economies				
		(million tons)		
Food	303.7	409.3	474.5	547.2
Feed	35.6	60.9	78.6	101.9
Other uses	46.4	64.1	75.4	88.5
TOTAL	385.7	534.3	628.5	737.6
		(kilograms)		
Per capita	220	233	240	246
Developing centrally planned economies				
		(million tons)		
Food	164.1	200.5	215.2	225.3
Feed	15.3	38.7	48.7	61.4
Other uses	24.6	32.6	36.0	39.1
TOTAL	204.0	271.8	299.9	325.8
		(kilograms)		
Per capita	257	290	298	304

*FAO projections based on "trend" GDP growth and U.N. "medium" population projections.

SOURCE: Overseas Development Council (1977) The United States and World Development Agenda. New York: Praeger Publishers, p. 184; adapted by the ODC from: Food and Agriculture Organization of the U.S. (1975) Population, Food Supply and Agricultural Development. Rome: FAO, p. 28.

TABLE 2 Food production indices (1961-65=100)

	1950 Total	1950 Per capita	1960 Total	1960 Per capita	1965 Total	1965 Per capita	1975 Total	1975 Per capita	1976 Total	1976 Per capita
HIGH-INCOME COUNTRIES	72	84	95	99	104	102	129	115	134	118
United States	76	94	97	101	106	103	136	120	138	121
Canada	82	113	92	97	112	108	128	106	142	116
Japan	68	79	97	100	103	101	115	100	109	94
Australia	65	87	89	95	99	95	139	113	130	104
European Community	69	77	95	98	103	101	121	112	118	109
DEVELOPING COUNTRIES	63	85	91	98	104	101	144	107	149	108
Poorest countries*	68	88	95	102	100	96	137	104	138	105
Bangladesh	74	101	95	102	106	101	127	95	129	94
Benin	73	95	102	109	100	95	119	87	121	86
Burma	37	48	91	97	98	94	117	91	120	91
Burundi	103	131	102	108	111	106	131	112	130	108

Poorest countries (Cont'd)

Ethiopia	78	98	93	99	104	100	105	79	109	80
Guinea	78	93	101	106	101	98	136	107	137	106
Haiti	92	113	100	105	99	99	104	84	107	84
India	65	80	95	101	96	92	139	108	139	106
Indonesia	59	80	100	108	102	97	156	118	157	116
Kenya	66	98	93	102	101	95	142	97	140	93
Madagascar	61	77	85	90	105	101	138	107	134	102
Malawi	63	83	86	88	116	136	175	123	170	117
Mali	85	108	98	104	97	93	88	68	94	71
Niger	61	88	82	92	108	102	87	62	98	69
Pakistan	77	108	85	92	110	104	163	115	168	115
Rwanda	59	81	101	108	101	96	148	107	148	104
Sierra Leone	76	95	93	98	101	97	134	102	137	102
Sri Lanka	56	78	87	93	87	83	108	83	99	75
Sudan	66	88	86	92	101	97	151	117	155	117
Tanzania	73	98	89	96	104	99	130	95	136	97
Uganda	90	130	90	98	113	107	107	74	105	70
Upper Volta	60	75	91	97	110	105	95	72	91	68
Zaire	104	143	109	118	106	101	146	110	150	110

TABLE 2 (Continued)

	1950 Total	1950 Per capita	1960 Total	1960 Per capita	1965 Total	1965 Per capita	1975 Total	1975 Per capita	1976 Total	1976 Per capita
Middle-income countries	60	84	89	97	107	101	148	107	155	109
Angola	78	95	95	100	104	101	87	72	80	65
Argentina	74	93	84	88	97	95	126	108	135	114
Bolivia	69	93	101	109	113	106	129	93	135	95
Brazil	59	85	87	95	115	109	164	117	181	126
Cameroon	83	104	92	97	111	107	120	97	121	96
Chile	78	106	97	105	107	102	132	103	136	105
Costa Rica	80	129	98	110	108	101	186	131	190	131
Cyprus	58	68	64	64	128	126	139	127	146	132
Colombia	69	104	92	102	107	101	160	116	166	118
Ecuador	38	56	90	99	106	101	152	108	149	103
Egypt	65	89	92	99	103	98	132	99	138	101
El Salvador	76	111	98	108	106	99	172	115	176	114
Ghana	57	79	91	98	99	94	122	89	123	87
Guatemala	65	95	89	99	105	98	191	139	207	146
Guyana	55	77	94	101	107	102	109	84	101	76
Honduras	75	112	90	99	109	102	103	68	125	80
Iran	47	66	88	96	105	99	171	121	179	122
Iraq	34	49	89	98	107	100	111	75	139	91
Ivory Coast	18	28	88	98	106	99	187	123	196	125
Jamaica	65	79	91	95	106	102	84	70	85	70

Middle-income countries (Cont'd)

Jordan	30	41	42	46	122	115	72	48	103	66
Korea, Republic of	56	74	81	89	110	104	154	116	168	124
Lebanon	55	77	73	79	110	104	146	105	149	105
Liberia	80	102	96	104	107	101	138	96	145	98
Libya	20	32	77	86	127	118	216	133	212	125
Malaysia (West)	59	82	88	95	110	104	238	173	265	188
Mexico	51	77	82	91	115	108	165	110	162	104
Morocco	67	93	101	108	117	112	118	85	154	107
Nicaragua	75	109	75	81	109	103	166	119	165	115
Nigeria	72	97	93	100	105	100	121	89	125	89
Panama	72	106	83	91	119	112	148	105	155	107
Paraguay	76	104	92	100	108	102	123	89	134	94
Peru	71	96	89	94	102	97	119	84	125	85
Philippines	38	56	89	97	109	103	161	113	173	118
Senegal	59	81	89	97	114	108	137	98	135	94
Syria	66	94	55	61	100	94	133	90	129	85
Thailand	63	89	86	93	103	97	170	120	168	116
Togo	67	88	101	108	110	105	131	98	133	97
Trinidad & Tobago	77	107	102	107	104	101	76	62	96	77
Tunisia	84	106	117	123	108	104	218	168	206	155
Turkey	55	79	95	103	103	98	148	110	153	111
Uruguay	80	96	91	95	109	108	109	104	129	122
Venezuela	47	76	89	99	115	108	172	117	165	109
Zambia	68	96	96	105	120	113	204	143	206	140

*Other "poorest" countries for which data were not available: Botswana, C.A.R., Chad, Gambia, Lesotho, Somolia, 2 Yemens, Afghanistan, Bhutan, Maldive Islands, Sikkim, Nepal, Laos, and West Samoa.

SOURCE: U.S. Department of Agriculture, Economic Research Service (1977).

Methodology for Establishing Research Priorities

The research priorities recommended in Chapter 2 were established in three overlapping phases covering a year, starting in February 1976. These three phases involved study teams covering 12 subject areas, a separate panel to rank the priorities recommended by the study teams, and the Steering Committee, respectively.

The overall task was to identify areas of research that would probably have the greatest effect on reducing worldwide hunger and malnutrition and that would probably produce earlier results if U.S. expenditures on them were increased. Each research area given priority was defined as a broad goal, such as increasing the amount of photosynthesis in major crops or reducing crop losses due to pests. Within these research areas, choices were made among lines of research that could advance such goals. At both levels, each research area considered is well above the individual project level.

The Study Team Phase

Twelve study teams, each covering a different subject, were established to select a group of high priority research areas within their subject matter scope. It was felt that the study teams would be the most productive in identifying and presenting the empirical and theoretical analysis needed to assess priorities. Assessment and ranking across subject matter research recommendations were done later by a separate

163

panel (Study Team 13). All of the study teams included both natural and social scientists, the balance depending on the subject area.

In examining possible research areas, each team addressed three questions posed by the Steering Committee:

1. What advances in knowledge will specific areas of research produce, and what is the scientific or technological significance of these advances?

2. If the research produces results, what effect would they likely have on reducing global hunger and malnutrition over the next several decades?

3. What supportive action will be required to conduct research for the accelerated activity recommended (e.g., more resources, policy changes, organizational changes)?

The study teams were asked to base their selection of research areas on their answers to the first two questions. Answers to the first and third questions provided insight on the feasibility of each research area. This information was used later by Study Team 13. These answers also provided raw material for Study Team 14 and the Steering Committee when they considered steps to mobilize and organize resources to implement the proposed research.

Each study team's selection of high priority research areas involved two steps. In the first step the study teams reviewed research recommendations and possibilities for research provided by existing reports, by the study team members themselves, and by other people who were consulted. The Steering Committee was particularly concerned that the study teams make full use of existing reports. From the hundreds of research possibilities, each team selected a limited set that would likely have the greatest global effect on hunger and nutrition. The second step further narrowed this set to research areas whose potential was thought to stand out well beyond that of the rest of the group.

On this basis, the 12 study teams selected over 100 research priorities. For each priority area they provided a statement, termed a research profile, of their responses to the three questions noted above. These profiles and the reports submitted by the study teams also included supplemental information in response to a series of subquestions posed by the Steering Committee (bearing on the three questions listed above), and other supporting information. The overall report and accompanying research profiles of each study team are published as the *Supporting Papers* for this report, together with the report of Study Team 14.

The Priority Ranking Phase

A separate panel, Study Team 13, had the task of making choices among the research areas selected as priorities by the study teams. Composed of 19 experts, broadly experienced in most aspects of food and nutrition, Study Team 13 assessed and ranked more than 100 research areas provided by the subject matter study teams.

This phase involved several steps:

- Study Team 13 and the Steering Committee staff discussed the scope, purpose, organization, and methods of the World Food and Nutrition Study and the process proposed for the study team's work.
- A staff group, including the lead analyst of Study Team 13, highlighted and annotated the full set of research priorities provided in profile form by the study teams. This procedure facilitated identifying the answers to the standard questions bearing on the selection of research priorities.
- The members of Study Team 13 then studied at length the annotated profiles and overview comments of the 12 study teams. They also met with each study team chairman, who highlighted his team's report and responded to questions.
- Next, each member of Study Team 13, without consulting with the others, ranked each research area from 0 to 10 according to four criteria: (1) probability of success, (2) global effect on hunger and malnutrition if the research succeeds, (3) cost and feasibility of doing the proposed research, and (4) overall priority, based on judgments about the first three criteria. Research areas were ranked according to these four criteria for two time periods: 15 years after the research effort is accelerated, and beyond 15 years. The key considerations for the overall priority rating were probability of success and effect. Feasibility moderated the decisions on how to do recommended research. Each member of Study Team 13 was requested to comment on all high or low ratings (8 to 10, 1 to 3). Each member also was invited to comment on any other point that he felt useful, such as interrelationships of priority areas, nature or appropriateness of assumptions, or gaps in needed analysis.
- The lead analyst of Study Team 13 and the Steering Committee staff summarized the rating sheets in three tables. The first table provided the average of Study Team 13's ratings on the eight criteria for each research area. The second table showed, for estimated effects in both less than and more than 15 years, the distribution of low, medium, and high *overall* ratings for each area, the ranking of the area's average

overall rating, and assignment of the research area to one of five priority categories based on the contents of the rating sheets and supplemental information in the profiles.

Those categories were:

A. High chance of successful research; very strong worldwide effect if research succeeds.

B. High chance of successful research; strong effect largely for specific geographic (political or ecological) zones or population groups.

C. Success of research relatively uncertain (more risky than A, B, or D, but chances still good); very strong worldwide effect if research succeeds.

D. High chance of successful research; relatively moderate effect if research succeeds (i.e., prospect of substantial global effect at low risk, though total effect of successful research well below A or C; effect could be more or less than B, but more diffused).

E. Lesser expectations than A to D.

The third table was an interpretive summary of the comments provided by the members of Study Team 13 on their rating sheets.

— Study Team 13 met to discuss the foregoing materials, especially research items on which there were highly divergent views, problems in dealing with uneven levels of scope and presentation among the research profiles, and difficulties in reaching conclusions in some subject areas on the basis of the materials at hand. During this period and also prior to the first ratings some items were combined into more comparable units.

— Study team members then provided a second round of individual ratings of a consolidated list of 76 research items. The ratings were confined to the overall priority of each research area, for effects in both the shorter and longer time periods. For this process, the study team members used their previous rating sheets, the research profiles, and the materials from the first two steps.

— Study Team 13 then prepared its report for the Steering Committee. It began by considering a list of all research items with an average rating in the second round above 6.0 in the short run and 7.0 in the long run. A list of items previously rated high, but not so high in the second rating, also was considered. The study team then discussed those items that ranked high and those areas in which there was concern that major omission or error might occur. Several items were added to the top priority list primarily to broaden and complete research areas. In addition, three areas of concern were identified that had no items in the top category, due to the study team's difficulties in dealing with the materials they received in the limited time available to them. The report identified 31 top priority and near top priority research areas for either short-run or long-run effect or both. The report also called attention to the need to develop priority research needs more adequately in three broad subject areas that Study Team 13 felt had been handled inadequately.

The Steering Committee Phase

Steering Committee staff and some Steering Committee members participated in the study team meetings. The staff provided procedural guidance and services for Study Team 13. The full Steering Committee began its participation in the priority assessment process in a two-day workshop with Study Team 13 (September 23–24, 1976). Discussion centered around a list of issues on the handling of priority selections for each of the subject areas covered by the first 12 study teams, including issues posed in the report of Study Team 13. Conclusions reached on these issues at the workshop, together with the report of Study Team 13 and the reports of the study teams, provided the basis for the first draft of Chapter 2 of the Steering Committee's report on research priorities. This involved some regrouping of priorities recommended by Study Team 13 and some filling in of gaps which Study Team 13 had identified.

At the workshop it was concluded that a special meeting was needed to develop adequate treatment of the policy and social science research area in the Steering Committee's report. An ad hoc group of Steering Committee and study team members met in mid-October. Working with a staff paper, this group resolved a number of issues and provided further guidance on this subject for the first draft of the Steering Committee report.

Another workshop was held December 15–17 to review and revise the first draft of the Steering Committee's report and to provide guidance for subsequent drafts. The Steering Committee and the chairmen or designated members of the 14 study teams attended. Some adjustments were made in the presentation of priorities in the course of a substantial recasting of the draft. Subsequent Steering Committee meetings and reworkings of the report over the following two months provided further adjustments in the presentation of research priorities.

The total process from September 1976 through to the final draft of the Steering Committee's report was influenced by comments and suggestions from members of the Board on Agriculture and Renewable

Resources (BARR) and of the Food and Nutrition Board of the Academy, and from many other persons who reviewed the study team reports and Steering Committee drafts. In particular, extensive individual and consolidated comments were received from BARR based on four reviews beginning with a workshop in August 1976 and carrying through reviews of Study Team 13 and Steering Committee drafts.

The International Rice Research Network

Achieving the research advances needed to meet their food production requirements in the decades ahead is beyond the capabilities of most if not all countries, and especially of the poorer and smaller countries. Moreover, it would not be economically or technically efficient to try to do so.

A practicable alternative is establishing systematic and continuing collaboration among national and international research organizations that are working on common or closely related problems. Arrangements for such collaboration are frequently called research "networks." By participating in such arrangements, countries with limited research capabilities in food and nutrition can draw on worldwide capabilities.

One of the best developed and most important examples of such a system of research is the international rice research network. Before delineating its operations, we should look briefly at how international agricultural research networks typically work.

Over the past decade there has been a sizable growth in international research networks concerned with food production. The informal structures of collaboration take advantage of possibilities for specialization and divisions of labor. The most important networks thus far involve research on the principal commodities consumed in the developing countries, such as rice, wheat, corn, cattle, sorghum, and cassava. But the same type of international cooperation is expanding for work on functional problems that extend across many commodities, such as design and use of fertilizers, soil and water management, pest control, and farming systems.

169

International agricultural research networks typically include institutions in developing countries, international research centers dealing with global or regional problems of developing countries, and research centers in high-income countries. Collaboration between institutions may take the form of joint research projects, pooling and exchanges of research materials and results (including stocks of genetic materials), program coordination, provision of research sites, advisory or training services, exchange visits, or use of common information services.

In these research networks, research collaboration follows the traditional pattern of voluntary cooperation among scientists or organizations sharing common interests. Initiatives and research products move in all directions through each system. However, the collaboration tends to be more extensive and systematic than the somewhat casual and intermittent international research collaboration that has long existed. One or more of the more advanced institutions in a network typically provide some "nerve center" functions that are needed for continuity of collaboration. These advanced institutions provide, for example, leadership in organizing programs or projects, logistical support, and information-management services.

Advanced research facilities, today mostly found in the high-income countries, are often relied on for the complex scientific and technological research required to solve basic problems; solutions at this level frequently have worldwide applications. The international research institutions usually provide model technology components or production systems that are widely usable, largely with adaptation, on a global or regional basis. Adaptation of technologies to national use and to specific farming situations normally is left to national research institutions. However, there are no hard and fast lines as to who does what. Each research organization (or scientist) in a research network, wherever located, can in principle contribute any relevant research results or services and can draw whatever it can use from the same pool.

The divisions of labor in the international research networks permit economies of scale by concentrating much of the more expensive and difficult types of research at facilities that can serve international needs, particularly the needs of developing countries. Widespread participation by developing countries in these networks permits testing solutions under a wide variety of ecological and socioeconomic circumstances, thereby speeding results and making them applicable over larger areas. This participation strengthens the abilities of researchers in developing countries or in international institutions to work in varied ecological settings and to bring home new insights and findings applicable to their own work. Tying U.S. research into the work of an appropriate network enhances the prospects for making U.S. research results effective at the farm level in developing countries.

Collaboration on Rice Research

Rice is the world's most important food crop. One and a third billion people—a third of the world's population—depend on rice for more than half of their calories and almost half of their protein. For another 400 million people rice is a major secondary staple, supplying 25 to 50 percent of their total calories. In some countries—Bangladesh, Burma, Khmer, Laos, Sarawak, Thailand, and Vietnam—rice supplies more than half of the protein consumed. Although most rice is produced and consumed in Asia, it is an increasingly important crop in the humid tropics of Latin America and Africa.

The regions heavily dependent on rice face a supply problem with three dimensions:

— Population increases in most rice-consuming countries are among the highest in the world. Consequently, demand for rice is expected to increase by at least 30 percent over the next decade alone, merely to maintain the current inadequate levels of consumption. Some countries that have traditionally exported rice are now having trouble producing enough food to feed their own expanding populations.
— The average annual income of those who depend primarily on rice is only about $80 to $90 per year. Since rice remains the preferred staple of the overwhelming majority, increases in per capita income will be transformed into greater demand for rice.
— Most arable land is already being farmed in the rice-growing nations so that most of the additional rice that is needed must be produced without bringing more land under cultivation. However, average rice yields in these nations are low, generally ranging between 1.2 and 1.8 tons per hectare in contrast to about 5 tons per hectare in the more developed countries.

Thus the problem is to accelerate the increase of rice yields over vast areas that are characterized by poverty and heavy population pressure on limited resources. The research and development requirements for adequate results, spanning dozens of different natural and socioeconomic environments, are beyond the individual capabilities of most if not all of the countries concerned.

To deal with this problem, a multifaceted system of research collaboration has been developed. The principal "nerve center" role is performed by the International Rice Research Institute, an autonomous international organization, originally established by the Ford and Rockefeller Foundations and now supported by 11 development assistance organizations. IRRI began its research operations in 1962 in the Philippines. In later years, international research institutes established in Latin America and Africa, with primary mandates in other research areas, undertook the responsibility for extending IRRI's results and capabilities in rice research and training in their regions. These institutes are the International Center for Tropical Agriculture (CIAT) in Colombia and the International Institute of Tropical Agriculture in Nigeria.

NETWORK ACTIVITIES LED BY IRRI

IRRI is involved in many types of collaboration with scientists and research organizations from the rice-growing countries of the world, including the high-income countries. These activities draw from and contribute to the research program that it carries out at its own facilities.

IRRI provides leadership and logistical, analytical, and materials services for five international collaborative programs. These activities are jointly planned, approved, and executed by researchers from the participating organizations, but IRRI scientists serve as catalysts and expediters and provide communication services.

First, in the International Rice Testing Program, standard sets of rice varieties obtained from IRRI and national research programs are tested and evaluated annually under a wide variety of agroclimatic conditions, using uniform procedures. The tests seek to improve a number of factors determining yield and stability of yield, and the results are shared by all participants. In 1976, these materials were tested at 475 locations in 50 rice-growing countries. Sixty-seven Asian scientists participated in international monitoring teams for this activity in Asia. The results guide further crossings and selections, which may be fed into subsequent worldwide testing programs.

Second, the International Rice Agroeconomic Network mobilizes teams of economists, agronomists, and other scientists who jointly evaluate the biological, physical, social, and economic factors influencing adoption of improved rice-growing technologies in order to guide research and policy work and to accelerate the beneficial effects of improved technology. In 1976, work proceeded according to jointly planned research agreements at 10 locations in six Asian countries.

Third, activities in the International Cropping Systems Network test combinations of genetically improved plants, equipment, and other physical innovations, and new farm production systems in cooperating countries, generally in large-scale pilot projects on farmers' fields. IRRI scientists and research and production personnel from each country collaborate in this effort. Different rice-based cropping patterns are tested under a variety of agroclimatic, soil, and socioeconomic conditions to develop the most appropriate combinations for each type of environment. The Masagana 99 experiment in the Philippines roughly doubled the annual yields of participating farmers using a new technology that permitted substituting two crops for one. In 1976, research and development was conducted at 21 sites in six Asian countries.

Fourth, in the Farm Machinery Development Network, IRRI is cooperating with national research organizations and manufacturers in developing mechanization appropriate for small farmers. In 1976, cooperative work was undertaken at 10 locations in eight countries. A number of the more successful machines are being manufactured by local firms in developing countries. These include a 5- to 7-horsepower tiller, small rotary weeder, small hand-propelled direct seeder, fertilizer applicator, 1-ton batch drier, and three small threshing machines.

The fifth collaborative research program is a specialized activity to develop rice varieties and associated technology for production under deepwater conditions. Work extends through Thailand, Bangladesh, India, Indonesia, Mali, and other countries.

IRRI also operates a comprehensive set of educational programs providing resident training for scientists and extension leaders from rice-producing nations. This includes a variety of research and production training, including two-week and six-month production courses, multiyear degree training in cooperation with various universities, and postdoctoral researchers and visiting scientists. From 1970 to 1974, an average of 143 participants were in residence for all or part of each year for training in research and production. Ninety percent of the trainees were from South and Southeast Asia, where most of the world's rice is grown. Other trainees came from Africa and Latin America, although most trainees from these continents are handled at IITA and CIAT. From 1962 to 1975, 1,055 people underwent intensive training at IRRI, and over a thousand more took IRRI's special two-week rice production course. The training provided through these programs can lead to subsequent research collaboration among the trainees and trainers and their research organizations.

IRRI further supports international research collaboration by promoting exchange of research results, ideas, and evaluation via symposia on technical problems, scientific publications, and its library services. Since its inception IRRI has organized 33 symposia, workshops, seminars, and conferences involving 1,760 scientists, mostly from national programs. Among IRRI's scientific publications are a detailed annual report of research results and other activities with a worldwide mailing list of 3,000; a newsletter sent to 5,300 rice scientists and research administrators; and an extensive bibliography of rice literature that is updated annually. There is an active documentation service at IRRI's headquarters in Los Banos, with a branch in Japan. The library tries to collect all documents on rice research and provides researchers with bibliographies on specialized subjects and information and photocopying services on request.

IRRI maintains a germ plasm bank that provides basic support for international genetic research to improve rice. The bank stores more than 35,000 seed varieties from every major rice-growing region of the world, contributed by and available to scientists throughout the world. Three to five thousand samples of seed are sent each year from the bank to cooperating scientists in national programs.

OTHER DIMENSIONS OF THE RICE RESEARCH NETWORK

CIAT and IITA conduct a range of research and development on rice with national and regional research organizations in Latin America and Africa that is similar in character to the IRRI pattern but of lesser scope. IRRI supports their rice work and has some direct involvements in these other regions; the centers arrange for interregional exchanges of experience. These activities led by the international centers in turn spark many arrangements for cooperation among national research programs.

Research collaboration among the various national and international research organizations in the developing countries occasionally uncovers situations in which lack of knowledge impedes the development of improved technologies. These situations call for scientific research that is beyond the capabilities of IRRI or other institutions in the rice research network or that can be pursued more efficiently in advanced research institutions that specialize in such problems. For example, IRRI is collaborating with the International Fertilizer Development Center in Alabama on improvement of fertilizers for rice production, with the Boyce Thompson Institute and Cornell University on biological nitrogen fixation, with Australian research organizations on drought tolerance, and with the International Center for Insect Physiology and Ecology in Kenya on pest problems. It also receives technical support from the International Board for Plant Genetic Resources on the handling and storage of the materials in its germ plasm bank.

The rice and wheat research networks are the most extensive and have had major international research programs established for long enough to have wide effects on world production. Two rough estimates of the international market value of increased wheat and rice production in 1972–73, which resulted from the use of new high yielding varieties generated in the rice and wheat networks, are $1.4 billion and $4 billion, respectively. In the two following years the use of improved rice varieties in 13 countries of Asia spread from 15.6 million hectares to 21.6 million hectares, or about 26 percent of their rice-producing area. IRRI is now leading collaborative research to deal with the needs of the nonirrigated rice areas bypassed by the early work, and with the disease and other stress and farming system problems that have limited wider use of higher yielding technologies.

Other Research Networks and the U.S. Role

In recent years, international research and development collaboration of the various types described above has been growing very rapidly in dozens of research fields that are important for U.S. and world food production. The arrangements for collaboration generally have much less scope and structuring than are found in the more mature rice, wheat, and corn networks, but a number of the newer networks are expanding. The international potato research program, for example, was set up on a network basis from the beginning and involves many institutions in the developing and high-income countries, including the United States.

U.S. institutions naturally are more active in commodity and subject areas in which we have developed particularly strong research activities for domestic reasons. Thus U.S. institutions have been much more involved in the international research collaboration on corn and wheat than on rice. In some subjects, U.S. institutions are beginning to play some of the "nerve center" roles described in the IRRI illustration. Title XII of the Foreign Assistance Act of 1975 has the potential to stimulate more of such activity. This international collaboration has brought important benefits for U.S. agriculture as well as providing opportunities to apply more U.S. research experience to the problems of the developing countries. The United States also has been instrumental in stimulating a new program of collaboration among the high-income countries that are members of the Organization for Economic Cooperation and Development on four basic food research problems of worldwide importance. This collaboration will include developing countries that are ready to participate as it gets under way.

A good start has been made in extending international research collaboration on world food and nutrition problems, but these activities are much stronger in the natural sciences than they are in the social sciences or in human nutrition. International research cooperation in the latter two areas needs much strengthening. The International Food Policy Research Institute, located in Washington, D.C., has the potential for playing some "nerve center" roles for portions of the needed international collaboration on social science research. The new United Nations University, located in Tokyo, might perform comparable functions for some of the needed collaboration on nutritional research and development since it is giving emphasis to this field in its start-up program.

APPENDIX

D

*Federal Agencies Affecting
the U.S. and World Food
and Nutrition Situation*

Approximately two dozen federal agencies have an influence on food supply and nutrition in the United States and the world. Half of these agencies conduct research on food and nutrition problems. Table 1 provides an estimate of the approximate level of expenditure on food and nutrition research by federal agencies.

The following descriptions are only indicative of the principal functions of federal agencies that affect the U.S. and world food and nutrition situation. The listing of functions is not complete.

U.S. Agencies that Conduct Research

DEPARTMENT OF AGRICULTURE

About half of the federal research on food and nutrition problems is financed and conducted by the U.S. Department of Agriculture (see Chapter 3). USDA has by far the most powerful influence of any agency on the U.S. and world food situations because of its leading role in setting policies for U.S. food production and marketing and for international trade in food, as well as its many programs and relationships with food producers, marketers, and consumers. About one-quarter of USDA's research funds are provided as matching grants to State Agricultural Experiment Stations (SAES), and USDA provides an organizational and leadership role for the overall USDA–SAES research community. USDA's

177

TABLE 1 Approximate level of expenditure on food and nutrition research by federal agencies*

Agency	Expenditure ($ million)
Department of Agriculture	360
Agency for International Development	69
National Institutes of Health (HEW)	60
National Science Foundation	40
Energy Research and Development Administration	45
National Oceanic and Atmospheric Administration (Commerce)	35
Department of the Interior	22
Environmental Protection Agency	15
Department of Defense	16
National Aeronautics and Space Administration	15
Tennessee Valley Authority	10
Food and Drug Administration (HEW)	3
Miscellaneous	10
TOTAL	700

*For the most part this information is not provided in regularly published data. Figures are based on informal estimates from departmental sources, relying on a mix of data for fiscal years 1975, 1976, and 1977.

role to date in nutrition research has been very modest ($13 million in fiscal year 1977).

AGENCY FOR INTERNATIONAL DEVELOPMENT

The Agency for International Development, a separate agency within the Department of State, has the primary responsibility within the U.S. government for international development assistance. AID's largest program, involving over half of its bilateral development assistance, is to foster food and nutrition improvements in developing countries. This includes a sizable and growing research component, which may reach perhaps $100 million or more by 1980, most of which involves U.S. research institutions in a variety of roles that are very supportive of what is done with much larger sums in the developing countries (see Chapter 3). Thus the effects of AID activities are felt both in the United States and around the world. AID supports research in both the natural and social sciences. As a major part of Title XII of the Foreign Assistance Act, AID is directed to expand and strengthen collaborative research efforts in food and nutrition involving U.S. universities, research institutions in the developing countries, and international research centers. The same act establishes a Development Coordinating Committee, which the

AID Administrator chairs, to coordinate all U.S. government policies that affect the developing countries.

DEPARTMENT OF HEALTH, EDUCATION, AND WELFARE

The largest federal expenditures for nutrition research are at the National Institutes of Health (see Chapter 3). The Food and Drug Administration conducts research and makes a broad range of regulatory decisions that have major effects on U.S. production, processing, and distribution of food, on the nutrition and health of our population, and on directions and scope of food research throughout the United States. Because of the growing U.S. foreign trade in food, these decisions increasingly affect what is done in foreign countries. NIH also supports a large amount of basic biological research outside the nutrition area that is important in building the scientific base for U.S. and worldwide advances in food production and consumer welfare.

NATIONAL SCIENCE FOUNDATION

The National Science Foundation makes research grants to U.S. scientists, primarily for projects in basic scientific fields. NSF's evolving mandate is carrying it increasingly into support of food-related and nutrition-related research, including basic work in the biological, social, and behavioral sciences, and applied research supported by the Research Applied to National Needs (RANN) program. This trend will probably continue. The authorizing legislation for NSF in fiscal year 1977 provides for increased support of international scientific collaboration on critical world problems such as food and nutrition. NSF also has a responsibility to help build U.S. capabilities for interdisciplinary research.

ENERGY RESEARCH AND DEVELOPMENT ADMINISTRATION

The decisions of the Energy Research and Development Administration (ERDA) on types of energy development affect all segments of the U.S. food system, from the seed to the kitchen. The same is true of its decisions affecting the allocation of scarce energy resources among competing uses. ERDA has been expanding its collaboration with USDA and its financial support for research on energy uses throughout the U.S. food system.

NATIONAL OCEANIC AND ATMOSPHERIC ADMINISTRATION

The National Oceanic and Atmospheric Administration, a separate agency within the Department of Commerce, manages oceanic and weather research and operations. It also participates in international programs and policy and regulatory negotiations on these matters, including ocean fisheries, the global activities of the National Marine Fisheries Service, and satellite and other technology applications.

DEPARTMENT OF THE INTERIOR

This agency makes decisions affecting land and water uses and reclamation in the United States for food production. The department conducts research on these areas, on vertebrate pests, and on other relevant areas. It also influences power generation and irrigation patterns, and plays the leading U.S. government role in aquaculture.

ENVIRONMENTAL PROTECTION AGENCY

The broad regulatory concerns and related research (about one-third of its budget) of the Environmental Protection Agency (EPA) will impinge increasingly on the means, costs, scope, and pattern of U.S. food production (and to some extent on AID programs). EPA is now focusing on reducing undesirable environmental effects of food production (mainly chemical pollution) and undesirable effects on food production of environmental pollution from other sources. Moreover, it makes general decisions on the production and use of toxic substances, sought for other reasons.

DEPARTMENT OF DEFENSE

The Defense Department (DOD) supports a strong food science research program, including work on nutrition and on dehydration, compression, and other means of preserving and concentrating food supplies. DOD plays an important role in the international movement of emergency food supplies. The Corps of Engineers influences irrigation and other water-use patterns. DOD develops and deploys sonar and other remote sensing technologies and facilities that have important potential for improving world food supplies. It supports social science and natural science research and intelligence work, some of which is relevant to improvement of food supplies in developing countries.

NATIONAL AERONAUTICS AND SPACE ADMINISTRATION

The National Aeronautics and Space Administration (NASA) conducts research and development on remote sensing for detection and monitoring of the earth's resources and supportive research in the life sciences. It collaborates in this work with USDA, AID, NOAA, and the U.S. Geological Survey. In the future satellites will play an increasingly important role in many aspects of the world food situation, including forecasting weather, estimating crops, and assessing and locating land and water availability and use potentials. Satellites will also be able to speed information exchange and other communications.

TENNESSEE VALLEY AUTHORITY

The Tennessee Valley Authority operates the largest research and development program in the world on chemical fertilizers. Its National Fertilizer Development Center is unique in this field. It is the primary source of research support for the U.S. fertilizer industry and its research and technical assistance services are widely used throughout the world, including the developing countries. The Center is now working with the new International Fertilizer Development Center, which gives TVA's research increased significance for developing countries.

Other Agencies with Important Policy Involvement

The following agencies have important program and policy responsibilities that affect the U.S. and world food and nutrition situation. However, their research role in this field is minor. This group does not include those agencies that primarily gather and assess data and other intelligence, such as the Central Intelligence Agency and the U.S. Geological Survey.

DEPARTMENT OF STATE (OTHER THAN AID)

The Department of State coordinates U.S. participation in international organizations, conferences, and negotiations affecting world food production and distribution. The State Department, the Department of Commerce, and other government agencies jointly establish policies on U.S. trade restrictions and promotion, and participate in related international negotiations that have an influence on world food production and trade patterns. The State Department, the Treasury Department, and other agencies play a similar role regarding international monetary policies (including exchange rates) and financial and development assistance, and in negotiations to establish or change international systems bearing on the rest of the world's production and consumption potentials. The Department of State also operates a major international intelligence and analysis network supporting these functions.

DEPARTMENT OF COMMERCE (OTHER THAN NOAA)

The Department of Commerce, along with USDA, Treasury, and other agencies, plays an important role in the international policy development affecting U.S. trade and investment and other international transactions described above in connection with the Department of State. The department has many programs of its own affecting international transactions that bear on the U.S. and world food production and trade patterns. It has important influences on internal U.S. trade in food and in agricultural inputs.

TREASURY DEPARTMENT

The Treasury Department shares a large part of the international role carried out by the State Department, and usually has leadership responsibility on financial matters. Its management of the U.S. revenue system and its role in shaping domestic fiscal and financial policies, including the role of credit and financial institutions, has important implications for the U.S. food and nutrition situation and U.S. participation in world food systems.

OTHER FINANCIAL POLICY INSTITUTIONS

The Export–Import Bank, the Federal Reserve Board, and other institutions affecting domestic and international lending patterns influence food systems. Recurrently, the United States establishes price stabilization and policy agencies of various types that share policy and control responsibilities with permanent agencies such as Treasury, the Office of Management and Budget, the Federal Reserve Board, and the Council of Economic Advisers. Strategies and decisions by these agencies can affect U.S. and world food trade and production patterns.

DEPARTMENT OF TRANSPORTATION

This department's policies, programs, and research support affect U.S. and international transport and storage systems for food.

DEPARTMENT OF LABOR

The influence of U.S. government policy on wages affects the relative costs of U.S. food supplies and their comparative international advantage.

OFFICE OF SCIENCE AND TECHNOLOGY POLICY

This new office within the Executive Office of the President is still being established. Two of the principal functions of the Office of Science and Technology Policy are to advise the President and Executive Branch on policies that will make the best use of U.S. scientific and technological capabilities, and to help coordinate U.S. research activities.

OTHER EXECUTIVE OFFICE AGENCIES

There are a number of coordinating and planning agencies within the Executive Office of the President that make policy decisions that indirectly affect the U.S. and world food situation. These include the Office of Management and Budget, the Council of Economic Advisers, the Domestic Council, and the National Security Council.

APPENDIX
E

Sources and Selected Bibliography

Sources

The principal sources of information used in preparing this study are mentioned below with indications of where and how they were used. In addition to published reports, a large amount of information and analysis was obtained directly from experts in the various relevant fields, and informal memoranda and unpublished reports, including reports of U.S. government agencies, were also obtained and used. The reports of the study teams provided the major input for the selection of research priorities, and also provided information that was useful in preparing other sections of the Steering Committee's report.

CHAPTER 1
Dimensions of the World Food and Nutrition Problem

Our discussion of the extent, nature, and incidence of malnutrition in the world draws heavily on assessments made by the Food and Agriculture Organization and the staff of the World Bank (also known as the International Bank for Reconstruction and Development). Analysis and data on nutritional status are presented in a number of FAO publications. These include the *Assessment of the World Food Situation: Present and Future,* prepared for the World Food Conference held in Rome in 1974; *The State of Food and Agriculture, 1975*; and the results of the Fourth World Food Survey published during 1976 in various issues of FAO's

Monthly Bulletin of Agricultural Economics and Statistics. A staff paper of the World Bank ("Malnutrition and Poverty," World Bank Staff Occasional Paper No. 23) also contains an estimate of the numbers of malnourished in the world.

The numbers of people suffering from malnutrition cannot be estimated precisely. However, the estimates made by FAO and the World Bank staff are certainly within a range of probable orders of magnitude and serve not only to underscore that large numbers of people in the developing world are affected by malnutrition, but also to provide a baseline against which our question, "What difference will it make if particular lines of research succeed?," can be measured.

FAO estimates the number of people suffering from malnutrition by comparing country and regional per capita requirements with estimates of per capita food supplies available. If per capita availabilities fall below requirements, malnutrition is assumed to exist. Additional supporting information on the incidence of malnutrition is derived from studies of energy intake by income or social group, vital statistics, clinical and anthropometric data, and detailed food-intake studies. Such data provide information on the nutritional status of children. The methodology used by FAO to estimate the extent of malnutrition is discussed in detail in the *Assessment of the World Food Situation* (pp. 53–74) and in *The State of Food and Agriculture, 1974* (pp. 103–110 and pp. 147–152).

World Bank staff estimates of the number of people who are malnourished are contained in "Malnutrition and Poverty." This report estimates the number of malnourished by relating nutritional status to income distribution. The methodology used by the World Bank is discussed on pages 11–25.

Data on population growth are from *Demographic Trends in the World and Its Major Regions, 1950–1970* and *Selected World Demographic Indicators by Countries, 1950–2000,* both prepared by the Population Division of the United Nations, the former for the World Population Conference held in Bucharest, August 1974. Additional information was made available by AID, the Bureau of the Census, and the Population Council.

We assume that there will be moderate and steady progress in reducing birth rates and rates of population increase to the year 2000 and beyond, and we have analyzed alternative rates of change that seem plausible based on published information. Any difference in these rates to the year 2000 would turn out to be rather inconsequential relative to the size of the food problem, basically because a large portion of the people to be fed are already born, as are most of the future mothers for the next 25 years, and because modification of the factors affecting net population change is likely to be slow. We expect a population of about 6 billion by 2000, but the recommendations in the report would not be changed by a figure well outside this.

The analysis of long-term trends in food production, consumption, trade and stocks, and of current supply and demand for food were based on materials prepared by the Economic Research Service and by the Foreign Agricultural Service of USDA. Other data sources include FAO's *Production Yearbook* and *Trade Yearbook*. The *World Food Situation and Prospects to 1985,* prepared by the Economic Research Service; analytical materials provided by the International Food Policy Research Institute; *A Hungry World: The Challenge to Agriculture,* prepared by the University of California; and the previously mentioned FAO *Assessment* were useful sources of information for our analysis of the dimensions and causes of the problem.

Data on per capita gross national product and country groupings by income class are from the *World Bank Atlas, 1976*; from *World Tables* (1976), prepared by the World Bank; and from AID.

CHAPTER 2
High Priority Research

In choosing priority areas for accelerated research, the Steering Committee was guided primarily by the subject matter reports of the study teams and by the report of Study Team 13 on priority assessment. The Steering Committee and the study teams used extensively a number of reports on food and nutrition research, particularly the *Interim Report* of the World Food and Nutrition Study and the accompanying report, *Enhancement of Food Production for the United States,* prepared by the Academy's Board on Agriculture and Renewable Resources, and the recommendations of the Food and Nutrition Board of the Academy's Assembly of Life Sciences. The study teams reviewed many other specialized studies in considering promising lines of research. A selected bibliography is given below. More extensive bibliographies can be found in the accompanying volumes of study team reports.

The report, *Agricultural Production Efficiency,* prepared by BARR in 1974, contains information that was considered in our selection of priorities. The report of the Agricultural Research Policy Advisory Committee (1976), *Research to Meet U.S. and World Food Needs,* also helped in the identification of research priorities.

Various government agencies supplied the Steering Committee with information on their research programs. The Steering Committee acknowledges the assistance of the U.S. Department of Agriculture, the

National Science Foundation, the Agency for International Development, the Department of State, the Department of Health, Education, and Welfare, and the National Oceanic and Atmospheric Administration.

Research priorities contained in the report of the Technical Advisory Committee to the Consultative Group on International Agricultural Research (1973), statements on international priorities from the directors of the international agricultural research centers and from Rockefeller Foundation staff, and reports of meetings considering particular research areas provided additional guidance in our consideration of promising areas of research.

Assessments of the potential benefits of research breakthroughs included in the discussion of each research area were prepared by the Steering Committee, using information from the study team reports, published studies, and standard data sources.

CHAPTER 3
How to Get the Work Done

In making its recommendations for action, the Steering Committee drew heavily on the report of Study Team 14, "Agricultural Research Organization."

USDA and state experiment station funding and data on scientist-years are also from Study Team 14, supplemented by USDA data and testimony presented to the Subcommittee on Science, Research and Technology and the Subcommittee on Domestic and International Scientific Planning and Analysis of the Committee on Science and Technology of the U.S. House of Representatives. Materials prepared by the Office of Technology Assessment on research expenditure for basic biological research were used in estimating present levels of funding and staff.

Recent levels of expenditure for international and U.S. assistance agencies are taken from annual budgets in the case of the World Bank and CGIAR, and from Congressional budget submissions for AID. Congressional committee reports on the International Development and Food Assistance Act of 1975, in addition to AID memoranda and analyses by U.S. university groups, give insight into the potential of Title XII, which provides for more effective involvement of U.S. universities in agricultural development assistance, including assistance in research, teaching, and extension.

Research expenditures by other federal agencies are from several sources, including the estimates prepared for the House Committee on Science and Technology and direct communications from the agencies involved.

Selected Bibliography

CHAPTER 1
Dimensions of the World Food and Nutrition Problem

Chenery, H., M. S. Ahluwalia, C. L. G. Bell, J. H. Duloy, and R. Jolly (1974) Redistribution with Growth. World Bank and the Institute of Development Studies, University of Sussex. London: Oxford University Press.

Food and Agriculture Organization of the U.N. (Selected Years) Production Yearbook. Rome: FAO.

Food and Agriculture Organization of the U.N. (Selected Years) Trade Yearbook. Rome: FAO.

Food and Agriculture Organization of the U.N. (Selected Years) Yearbook of Fishery Statistics. Rome: FAO.

Food and Agriculture Organization of the U.N. (1970) Indicative World Plan for Agriculture. Rome: FAO.

Food and Agriculture Organization of the U.N. (1974) Assessment of the World Food Situation: Present and Future. Document C/CONF. 65/3, World Food Conference. Rome: FAO.

Food and Agriculture Organization of the U.N. (1975) The State of Food and Agriculture, 1974. Rome: FAO.

Food and Agriculture Organization of the U.N. (1976) Monthly Bulletin of Agricultural Economics and Statistics. Vol. 25, nos. 4 and 7/8.

Food and Agriculture Organization of the U.N. (1976) The State of Food and Agriculture, 1975. Rome: FAO.

International Bank for Reconstruction and Development (1976) World Bank Atlas, 1976. Washington, D.C.: IBRD.

International Bank for Reconstruction and Development (1976) World Tables. Washington, D.C.: IBRD.

International Food Policy Research Institute (1976) Meeting Food Needs in the Developing World. Research Report No. 1. Washington, D.C.: IFPRI.

International Food Policy Research Institute (1977) Recent and Prospective Developments in Food Consumption: Some Policy Issues. Draft report prepared for the 24th session of the Protein Advisory Group (PAG) of the U.N., January 31–February 4, 1977.

International Labor Office (1976) Employment, Growth and Basic Needs: A One-world Problem. Geneva: ILO.

Johnson, D. G. (1975) World Food Problems and Prospects. Washington, D.C.: American Enterprise Institute for Public Policy Research.

National Research Council (1975) Population and Food: Crucial Issues. Report of the Committee on World Food, Health, and Population, Division of Biological Sciences, Assembly of Life Sciences. Washington, D.C.: National Academy of Sciences.

Overseas Development Council (1977) The United States and World Development Agenda 1977. New York: ODC/Praeger Publishers.

Reutlinger, S. and M. Selowsky (1976) Malnutrition and Poverty. World Bank Staff Occasional Paper No. 23. Washington, D.C.: IBRD.

United Nations, Population Division (1974) Demographic Trends in the World and Its Major Regions, 1950–1970. E/CONF. 60/CBP 14. New York: U.N.

United Nations, Population Division (1975) Selected World Demographic Indicators by Countries, 1950–2000. ESA/P/WP.55. New York: U.N.

U.S. Agency for International Development (1975) GNP: Growth Rates and Trends, 1974. Washington, D.C.

U.S. Department of Agriculture (Selected Years) Agricultural Statistics. Washington, D.C.: U.S. Government Printing Office.

U.S. Department of Agriculture (1974) The World Food Situation and Prospects to 1985. Foreign Agricultural Economic Report No. 98, Economic Research Service. Washington, D.C.: U.S. Government Printing Office.

U.S. Department of Agriculture (1976) The World Agricultural Situation. Economic Research Service. Washington, D.C.

U.S. Department of Agriculture (1976) World Fertilizer Review. Economic Research Service. Washington, D.C.

University of California Food Task Force (1974) A Hungry World: The Challenge to Agriculture. Berkeley: University of California.

CHAPTER 2

High Priority Research

Berg, A., N. S. Scrimshaw, and D. L. Call, eds. (1971) Nutrition, National Development and Planning: Proceedings of an International Conference. Cambridge, Massachusetts.

Brown, A. W. A., T. C. Byerly, M. Gibbs, and A. San Pietro (1975) Crop Productivity: Research Imperatives. East Lansing, Michigan: Michigan State Agricultural Experiment Station and Charles F. Kettering Foundation.

Consultative Group on International Agricultural Research, Technical Advisory Committee (1974) Priorities for International Support to Agricultural Research in Developing Countries. Rome: FAO.

Cornell University (1976) Potential Increases in Food Supply Through Research in Agriculture. Ithaca, New York.
  —Fertilizers and Increased Food Production
  —Food Science Research and Nutritive Value of Food Products
  —Research Needs on Pesticides and Relative Problems for Increased Food Supplies
  —Researchable Areas Which Have Potential for Increasing Crop Production
  —Constraints on Increasing Agricultural Production in the Tropics: Research and Implementation Needs
  —Increased Productivity from Animal Agriculture

Cramer, H. H. (1967) Plant Protection and World Crop Production. Leverkusen, Federal Republic of Germany: Farbenfabriken Bayer A.G.

Dvoskin, D. and E. Heady (1976) Economic and Environmental Impacts of Energy Rationing in Agricultural Production. Ames, Iowa: Iowa State University.

Dunn, E. S. (1974) Social Information Processing and Statistical Systems: Change and Reform. New York: Wiley and Sons.

Eckholm, E. (1976) Losing Ground; Environmental Stress and World Food Prospects. New York: Norton.

Esmay, M. L. and C. W. Hall, eds. (1973) Agricultural Mechanization in Developing Countries. Tokyo: Shin-Norinsha Company, Ltd.

Evans, H. J., ed. (1975) Enhancing Biological Nitrogen Fixation. Washington, D.C.: National Science Foundation.

Food and Agriculture Organization of the U.N. (1974) The World Food Problem: Proposals for National and International Action. Document E/CONF. 65/4, World Food Conference. Rome: FAO.

Harrison, K., D. Henley, H. Riley, and J. Shaffer (1974) Improving Food Marketing Systems in Developing Countries: Experiences from Latin America. Research Report No. 6. Latin American Studies Center, Michigan State University, East Lansing.

Iowa State University (1977) Proceedings, World Food Conference of 1976. Ames, Iowa: Iowa State University Press.

Massachusetts Institute of Technology, Department of Nutrition and Food Science (1976) Protein Resources and Technology: Status and Research Needs. Cambridge, Massachusetts.

Mukhijani, A. (1975) Energy and Agriculture in the Third World. Cambridge, Massachusetts: Ballinger Publishing Company.

National Research Council (1972) Genetic Vulnerability of Major Crops. Washington, D.C.: National Academy of Sciences.

National Research Council (1975) Agricultural Production Efficiency. Washington, D.C.: National Academy of Sciences.

National Research Council (1975) Enhancement of Food Production for the United States. Washington, D.C.: National Academy of Sciences.

National Research Council (1975) More Water for Arid Lands. Board on Science and Technology for International Development, Commission on International Relations. Washington, D.C.: National Academy of Sciences.

National Research Council (1975) Pest Control: An Assessment of Present and Alternative Technologies. Washington, D.C.: National Academy of Sciences.

National Research Council (1975) Recommendations on Nutrition Research and Development. Food and Nutrition Board, Assembly of Life Sciences. Washington, D.C.: National Academy of Sciences.

National Research Council (1975) Understanding Climatic Change: A Program for Action. U.S. Committee for the Global Atmospheric Research Program. Washington, D.C.: National Academy of Sciences.

National Research Council (1976) Climate and Food. Report of the Committee on Climate and Weather Fluctuations. Washington, D.C.: National Academy of Sciences.

Office of Technology Assessment (1975) Food, Agriculture and Nutrition Information Systems. Washington, D.C.

Orvedal, A. C. and K. T. Ackerson (1972) Agricultural Soil Resources of the World. U.S. Department of Agriculture, Washington, D.C.

President's Science Advisory Committee (1967) The World Food Problem. Washington, D.C.: U.S. Government Printing Office.

Shumway, C. R. (1973) Allocation of Scarce Resources to Agricultural Research: Review of Methodology. American Journal of Agricultural Economics 55:557–566.

U.S. Agency for International Development (1973) AID Research 1971–1973. Washington, D.C.

U.S. Department of Agriculture (1976) Research to Meet U.S. and World Food Needs. Report from conference held July 7–9, 1975 in Kansas City, Missouri. Agricultural Research Policy Advisory Committee, Washington, D.C.

Ward, D. J. and H. R. Fortmann (1976) A National Program of Agricultural Energy Research and Development: A Report to the National Planning Committee of the Agricultural Research Policy Advisory Committee. Washington, D.C.

CHAPTER 3
How to Get the Work Done

Arndt, T. M., D. G. Dalrymple, and V. W. Ruttan, eds. (1977) Resource Allocation and Productivity in National and International Agricultural Research. Minneapolis: University of Minnesota Press.

Boyce, J. K. and R. Evenson (1975) National and International Agricultural Research and Extension Programs. New York: Agricultural Development Council.

Consultative Group on International Agricultural Research (1977) Report of the Review Committee. Washington, D.C.

Evenson, R. E. and Y. Kislev (1975) Agricultural Research and Productivity. New Haven: Yale University Press.

Long, R. W. and G. Bentley (1975) Joint Statement Presented to Subcommittee on Science, Research and Technology and on Domestic and International Scientific Planning and Analysis of the House Committee on Science and Technology. Washington, D.C.

Moseman, A. H. (1970) Building Agricultural Research Systems in the Developing Nations. New York: Agricultural Development Council.

National Research Council (1974) African Agricultural Research Capabilities. Washington, D.C.: National Academy of Sciences.

Rockefeller Foundation (1974 and 1976) Strategies for Agricultural Education in Developing Countries. Reports of the First and Second Bellagio Conferences. New York, New York.

U.S. House of Representatives (1976) Special Oversight Review of Agricultural Research and Development. Report by the Subcommittee on Science, Research and Technology and the Subcommittee on Domestic and International Scientific Planning and Analysis. Washington, D.C.: U.S. Government Printing Office.